THE ALZHEIMER'S PROJECT

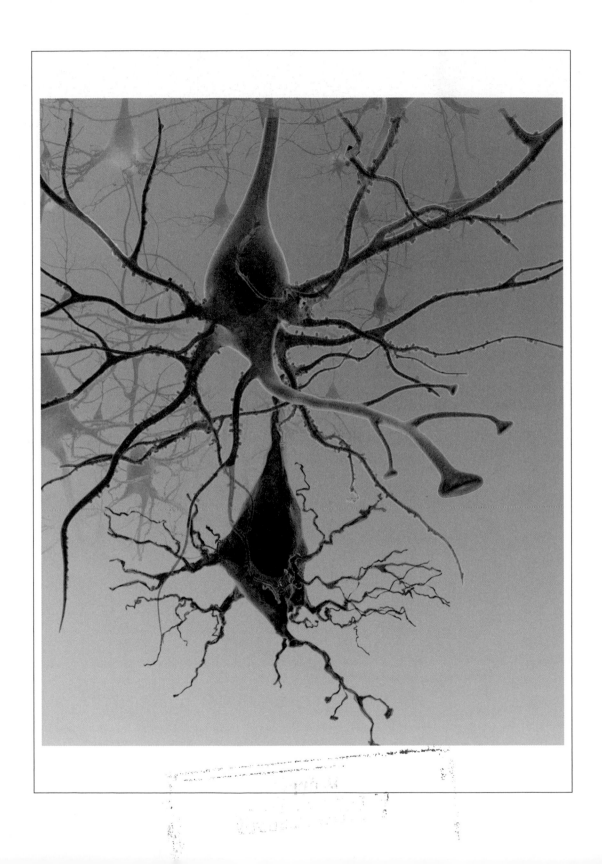

THE
ALZHEIMER'S
PROJECT

MOMENTUM IN SCIENCE

JOHN HOFFMAN AND SUSAN FROEMKE
WITH SUSAN K. GOLANT

BASED ON THE HB⊙ DOCUMENTARY

PRESENTED BY

HBO Documentary Films and the National Institute on Aging of the National Institutes of Health

IN ASSOCIATION WITH THE

Alzheimer's Association®, Fidelity® Charitable Gift Fund℠, and Geoffrey Beene Gives Back® Alzheimer's Initiative

Contributing writer: Alexandra Moss
Science consultant: Anne Brown Rodgers

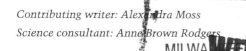

Developed by Book Tree

PublicAffairs NEW YORK

Illustration opposite the title
page compares a healthy neuron
(above) to one damaged by
Alzheimer's disease (below).

Book developer: Alison Brown Cerier
Copyeditor: Jane Cavolina
Published in the United States by PublicAffairs™, a member of the Perseus Books Group.

Book Design by Jenny Dossin.

Library of Congress Cataloging-in-Publication Data
Hoffman, John, 1959-
    The Alzheimer's project : momentum in science / John Hoffman and Susan Froemke with Susan K. Golant. —1st ed.
        p. cm.
    "Based on the HBO documentary presented by HBO Documentary Films and the National Institute on Aging of the National Institutes of Health in association with the Alzheimer's Association, Fidelity Charitable Gift Fund, and Geoffrey Beene Gives Back Alzheimer's Initiative."
    Includes index.
    ISBN 978-1-58648-756-0 (hardcover)
    1. Alzheimer's disease. 2. Health education. I. Froemke, Susan. II. Golant, Susan K. III. Title.
    RC523.H64 2009
    616.8'31—dc22
                                                                                    2009010293

First Edition
10 9 8 7 6 5 4 3 2 1

CONTENTS

FOREWORD

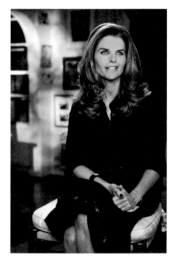

I've been a child of Alzheimer's disease since my father, Sargent Shriver, was diagnosed in 2003. When a loved one is diagnosed with Alzheimer's disease, it affects the entire family, and it affects each member differently.

In the first years of my father's illness, I approached the disease not only as the daughter of someone who has it, but also as the mother of children who have to deal with it, too. I struggled to find a way to give my four kids a real sense of what a special man their grandfather was and to help them understand what this disease was doing to him.

That struggle resulted in my third children's book, *What's Happening to Grandpa?* It was a way for me to share the questions my children and my nieces and nephews were asking about my dad and give them answers they could understand and internalize. I hoped it would also help the millions of others dealing with this disease. Writing about Alzheimer's disease helped me, too, because my father has always been such a cheerful and positive person, and I wanted the book to reflect how that attitude lit up his life and ours.

In truth, my children's questions and concerns also provoked my own anxieties. What were my chances of developing the disease, I wondered? Were there things I could do to prevent it? Were there drugs I could take? Was there something out there that could help my dad and help him now? If not, why not? I learned that there were, in fact, medications that helped maintain his cognitive abilities early on, but the effect lasted only so long. Since then, there's been no medication to stave off his continuing decline.

Participating in *The Alzheimer's Project* has allowed me to explore the answers to all my questions in much more depth than I ever imagined. As an executive producer of the project, I've learned how far scientists have come in figuring out the genetic and environmental causes of the disease, imaging the earliest signs of it in the brain, understanding the disease process, and working to develop drugs that could potentially delay its onset or prevent it altogether.

I had the privilege of joining HBO on some of their shoots with scientists at the forefront of these discoveries. I met Dr. Charles De-Carli, a neurologist at the University of California Davis, who is looking into the connection between vascular disease and Alzheimer's disease. I visited a lab at the University of California Irvine, where Dr. Carl Cotman is researching how exercise and diet may keep the ravages of Alzheimer's disease at bay and allow us to age more healthfully. I got to enter the futuristic world of biotech innovation in the Bay Area, where Dr. Dale Schenk showed me the promising work he's conducting on a potential vaccine for Alzheimer's disease at Elan Pharmaceuticals. As the first lady of California, I'm proud that so much of the trailblazing research is going on in our state.

My father was a great proponent of public service. In the course of his own career in government, he helped found the Peace Corps, Head Start, Job Corps, Legal Services for the Poor, and countless other programs that up to the present day help people who are struggling to live above the poverty line. I believe scientists focusing on Alzheimer's disease are also performing public service of the highest order. Today, our federal government, through the National Institutes of Health, does enormous public good by funding and conducting one of the world's most extensive Alzheimer's disease research programs. Foundations such as the Alzheimer's Association also play an important role. I've come to believe that scientific research is one of the most important investments our government can make—scientific research that may one day produce treatments and prevention strategies, so that fewer families will have to go through what my family has gone through because of Alzheimer's disease.

I also firmly believe that each and every one of us can play a role in finding a cure. We can walk to raise money. We can visit people in Alzheimer's disease homes and read to them, play music for them, or just visit. Of course, it's hard to say what's going on in the mind of someone with Alzheimer's disease. But we all know what's going on in our own hearts when we feel loved. It feels good. Letting people with Alzheimer's disease know they're still loved might not bring back all the memories they once had—but I know in my own heart it can bring them the comfort of remembered love.

MARIA SHRIVER

RESPONDING TO THE CHALLENGE

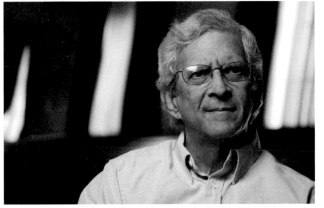

When HBO producers John Hoffman and Susan Froemke came to us at the National Institute on Aging about contributing our scientific expertise to a large-scale public health outreach project on Alzheimer's disease, we gave a great deal of thought to how to approach it. We are working very hard on the prevention and treatment of Alzheimer's disease and have made enormous strides in understanding its origins and developing potential routes for prevention and therapy. However, research has yet to achieve success, as defined by the ability to prevent Alzheimer's disease or, if it develops, to slow its progression. Although the research challenge remains significant, there is a very important, informative, and compelling story to tell—about the dedication of all the scientists and families who are on the front lines of the fight against Alzheimer's disease and the progress we are making, and will make, together. It is, in a word, a story of hope.

In the three decades since the scientific study of Alzheimer's disease began in earnest, an increasingly productive research program has been established. It approaches the study of age-related cognitive change and dementia on several different fronts—the basic biology of the disease, genetic and non-genetic influences, drug development and clinical aspects, and approaches to caregiving. Today, innovative technologies in imaging and genetics in particular are allowing exploration in ways we never imagined before. And we have a well-developed infrastructure of academic research centers and consortia to carry out this critical work. What we've learned is generating new excitement about the potential for intervening and making a difference in the disease.

Our efforts come none too soon. The world's population is aging at an accelerating rate, a critical trend because aging is the best established risk factor for Alzheimer's disease. Studies indicate that the probability of developing the disease doubles every five years after age sixty-five. Among people age eighty-five and older, as many as half may suffer from Alzheimer's disease. The baby boomers, the first of whom reaches that milestone sixty-fifth birthday in 2011, will soon be entering the ages of increasing risk. In sheer numbers, the statistics are daunting. In 2000, thirty-five million people were older than sixty-five. By 2050, according to one census estimate, the number of older people will double, led by growth in the numbers of people age eighty-five and older, those at most risk for Alzheimer's disease.

These demographics press the urgency to address Alzheimer's disease. The first concern is the human toll for the greater number of people who will develop the disease and, with it, an increase in the ranks of caregivers. Add the financial and broader societal burden, and the costs will simply be unsustainable if we fail over the next twenty years to reduce the risk to older people. In dollar terms, it is estimated that the direct and indirect costs of Alzheimer's disease in the United States today are at least one hundred billion dollars annually, including medical care, caregiving, and lost productivity.

We cannot predict exactly how and when we will turn the corner to find a truly effective intervention against Alzheimer's disease. But I can report that enormous progress in understanding the disease is leading to development of experimental drugs and to clinical testing of a number of compounds. We have learned much about the complexity of factors involved in Alzheimer's disease. But there is also new thinking about how to address the combination of genetic and environmental influences that may put us at risk or, conversely, might protect us from developing dementia.

One of the most rapidly moving areas of research is genetics, examining the most basic influences on our health. Our genes direct the production of proteins that make up body structures like organs and tissue, as well as controlling chemical reactions and carrying on signaling between cells. A first step in determining the start of any disease process is pinpointing relevant genes and genetic mutations.

Over the past few decades, we have discovered some of the genetic clues to Alzheimer's disease. Three genetic mutations are responsible for causing a very rare, early-onset form of the disease, which accounts mostly for cases that occur under age sixty. For late-onset disease, in those aged sixty-five and older, which affects the vast majority of people with Alzheimer's disease, the genetic picture is much less clear. In these cases, genes may increase the risk of Alzheimer's disease, but no single gene has been shown to directly cause disease. One gene, apolipoprotein E (ApoE), is such a risk factor for late-onset Alzheimer's disease, with one form of the gene appearing more often in people with Alzheimer's disease than in those without. It is likely that other genes are in this class of risk factors.

Today, a major search effort is under way to find additional genetic associations for Alzheimer's disease. To do so, scientists must compare data from thousands of people who have the disease with data from people who do not have it, to see whether there are particular genetic correlations. To expand and accelerate discovery, the National Institute on Aging launched the Alzheimer's Disease Genetics Initiative, which brings together investigators at multiple centers to conduct highly sophisticated genetic analyses on at least one thousand families. In 2008, the Alzheimer's Disease Genetics Consortium was established to take advantage of new technologies for genome-wide association studies. That effort involves rapidly scanning markers across the complete sets of DNA, or genomes, of many people to find genetic variations associated with the disease. Data from both of these projects will be shared with qualified investigators for further analysis.

The discoveries from these initiatives should provide important clues to the Alzheimer's disease process and, ultimately, reveal potential targets for drugs and other interventions.

Armed with knowledge of basic disease processes already gained from genetic insights and the study of factors like protein conformation, inflammation, and oxidative stress, we know about important fundamentals of the Alzheimer's disease process and how it damages and ultimately destroys brain cells and communications. We have aimed our sights squarely at one of the best-developed areas of research thus far, the formation of the beta-amyloid plaques characteristic of Alzheimer's disease, which are formed by fragments of a larger protein found in brain cells and which interfere with how neurons talk to one another. We have also discovered that the tangles in the brains of people with Alzheimer's disease, the second hallmark pathology of the disease, are made up of the protein tau, whose normal role in supporting cell structures is compromised.

As we peer deeper at the molecular and cellular level, what other factors could influence our chances of getting Alzheimer's disease? A great deal of evidence from large-scale epidemiological studies suggests that the factors affecting heart health, such as blood pressure, cholesterol, and blood glucose, may overlap with the risk and protective factors for brain health and function. These include observations that link exercise, maintaining a healthy weight, and controlling blood pressure in midlife to a lower risk of developing Alzheimer's disease later in life. Studies in animal models also associate exercise and healthy diet with reduced risk of cognitive decline. Additional clinical trials of these interventions are being conducted in humans to determine definitively whether they reduce the risk of cognitive decline. But they are clearly important for controlling cardiovascular disease and diabetes, and so we recommend healthy lifestyle factors for both their known and potential benefits.

This productive portfolio of basic, epidemiological, animal, and clinical research has led to the development and testing of a number of potential interventions to prevent or delay the onset of Alzheimer's disease or slow its progression. The institute is also building a robust translational research program that supports the discovery and development of new treatments for Alzheimer's disease to the stage where they can be tested in clinical trials supported by the government or private sector. It is estimated that there are ninety-one new drugs in clinical trials. Overall, more than two hundred clinical trials of interventions are under way, including the testing of new drugs, natural products, and lifestyle interventions such as exercise. These studies involve thousands of individuals across the United States and are supported by both the public and the private sector.

Research in caregiving is finding better ways to manage care at home and in an institutional setting. This is a vital area of study for families now coping with the disease. Pilot testing is being done to see how the innovative REACH (Resources for Improving Alzheimer's Caregiver Health) program of successful interventions for caregivers might be adopted more widely. The effort involves over a dozen Department of Veterans Affairs programs around the United States (REACH-VA) and several statewide programs funded by the Administration on Aging.

Our progress so far—and prospects for the future—depends in important ways on coordination and collaboration among the research community, with the private sector, and across the government. The network of twenty-nine Alzheimer's Disease Research Centers supported by the National Institute on Aging undertake basic and clinical research as well as training, education, and the dissemination of technology, with a key function being the coordination of studies and sharing of data. The institute also manages the nation's foremost clinical trials network in this area, the Alzheimer's Disease Cooperative Study.

We recognize the importance of collaboration between the public and the private sector to advance research and knowledge. A model partnership is the Alzheimer's Disease Neuroimaging Initiative. This sixty-million-dollar multi-year project includes the government, academia, the Alzheimer's Association and Institute for the Study of Aging, and a number of pharmaceutical and imaging companies. It is designed to demonstrate how brain imaging techniques and biomarkers in blood and cerebrospinal fluid may be able to signal Alzheimer's disease before clinical symptoms appear. That would help detect the disease at its earliest stages, track progression, and monitor the effect of interventions. What we learn will enable us to conduct clinical trials more quickly and efficiently. Already, preliminary findings from this and other studies suggest that we can "see" Alzheimer's disease plaques in the living brain and that there may be markers for Alzheimer's disease, in the same way that cholesterol signals cardiovascular disease.

It is in the spirit of such collaborations that we at the National

Institute on Aging accepted HBO's invitation to provide scientific input and technical guidance for *The Alzheimer's Project*. As part of the National Institutes of Health at the U.S. Department of Health and Human Services, the institute has the leading responsibility in the United States government for research in Alzheimer's disease. Along with our sister NIH institutes and centers and other federal agencies, including the Administration on Aging, with its interest in caregiver research and support, and the Food and Drug Administration, which evaluates the safety and efficacy of new drugs and devices used in diagnosis and treatment, we are the taxpayers' primary investment in Alzheimer's disease programs. As such, it is the National Institute on Aging's mission, in addition to research, to report on research progress and to promote understanding of science and health with respect to aging and Alzheimer's disease.

I am pleased that we have been able to work with the Alzheimer's Association, Fidelity Charitable Gift Fund, and the Geoffrey Beene Gives Back Alzheimer's Initiative, in collaboration with HBO's Sheila Nevins and John Hoffman, and with Executive Producer Maria Shriver, to provide a front-row seat at the laboratory bench. We dedicate our efforts to the millions of people touched by Alzheimer's disease—those supporting research, those participating in studies, and, especially, those with Alzheimer's disease and their families and friends.

DR. RICHARD J. HODES
Director, National Institute on Aging
National Institutes of Health
U.S. Department of Health and Human Services

THE MAKING OF

THE ALZHEIMER'S PROJECT: MOMENTUM IN SCIENCE

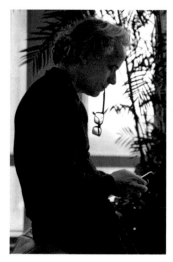

Through the experience of producing *The Alzheimer's Project: Momentum in Science,* I lost my fear of developing the disease.

This was not the first time I was confronted with the prospect of producing a campaign on Alzheimer's disease. Ten years ago my father, Emanuel Hoffman, died of the disease at the age of eighty. Manny was a newspaper journalist and editor and his decline into dementia was long and slow. My father's illness frightened me as much it saddened me. Would I share his fate? Was his father's, my grandfather's, senility just another word for the same condition? A short while after his death, Sheila Nevins, the president of HBO Documentary Films, asked if I thought the time was right to do a film on Alzheimer's disease. My gut reaction was to say no. I had a difficult time considering the notion of spending two years immersed in the disease that destroyed my father. The truth was, I was terribly reluctant to learn more about it. Over the course of my father's illness and well beyond his death, I was filled, right or wrong, by a pervasive sense of hopelessness about Alzheimer's disease.

Two years ago, I was forced to confront my fears of Alzheimer's again after HBO premiered *The Addiction Project,* and we began our search for the next public health campaign for HBO to produce. *The Addiction Project* was a considerable HBO–National Institutes of Health effort to educate the American public about advances in the understanding of addiction as a treatable brain disease. We conveyed life-changing information to more than fifty million Americans via a wide array of media platforms. With this success, Sheila Nevins asked me and Susan Froemke (my producing partner) to return to the NIH. As a pay cable network, HBO has an invitation into thirty million homes and, when all cable households are invited to watch certain events for free, that audience grows to as many as one hundred million homes. It's important to recognize Sheila's and HBO's belief that such reach must sometimes be used for public health purposes. After *The Addiction Project,* Susan's and my task was to explore other ways we could combine the medical and scientific expertise of the National Institutes of Health with the scope and excellence of HBO programming. The goal was to find a medical problem affecting millions of Americans for which science had made great advances of which the public was unaware. Where had the National Institutes of Health and the research community found hope for solving a disease where little hope was perceived? The resounding answer was Alzheimer's disease.

How was it that such advances in Alzheimer's research had escaped me? I read the *Science Times* avidly, I listen to NPR, I make science films! I had gradually taken my head out of the sand about this disease, yet I believed incorrectly that Alzheimer's disease research was still in its infancy, that the biggest controversy in the field revolved around the risks of cooking in aluminum pots (a long-disproved theory), and that the most I could do to minimize my chance of getting the disease was to solve crossword puzzles—which I do anyway.

I now know that I was not alone in my anxiety about developing Alzheimer's disease. According to a recent study, it is the second most feared illness among the general U.S. population, and it is the most feared illness among women. The baby boomers are seeing nearly 50 percent of their parents' generation struggle with Alzheimer's disease by the time they reach eighty-five, and in 2011 the first boomers will themselves reach retirement age, setting off a precipitous rise in the incidence of the disease, which already affects as many as five million Americans.

Through our collaboration with the National Institute on Aging (NIA) of the National Institutes of Health and the Alzheimer's Association, we achieved a remarkable level of access to the scientific community. The National Institutes of Health spend about half a billion dollars on Alzheimer's disease research each year, funding the work of the nation's greatest minds, who are applying their brilliance toward unraveling the genetics, neuroscience, pathology, prevention, and treatment of Alzheimer's disease. While the Alzheimer's Association has a smaller research funding profile, they do publish the definitive research journal *Alzheimer's & Dementia* and host the International Conference on Alzheimer's Disease. The seventy-two chapters of the Alzheimer's Association are the support lifeline for people with the disease and their families. Susan Froemke and I, along with our pair of dedicated young associate producers, Matt Heineman and Ali Moss, could not have become educated students of Alzheimer's disease without the support of these two organizations. And, of course, *The Alzheimer's Project* could not have grown to the level we've achieved without the support of the Geoffrey Beene Gives Back Alzheimer's Initiative and the Fidelity Charitable Gift Fund.

The chill I still felt at the mention of Alzheimer's disease began to dissipate in the spring of 2007 with our immersion in the science of Alzheimer's disease. We studied hundreds of research papers, journal articles, and, in particular, the National Institute on Aging's annual Progress Reports. We carefully examined twenty hours of taped presentations by a select gathering of scientists in Tübingen, Germany, recognizing the one hundredth anniversary of Dr. Alois Alzheimer's historic discovery of plaques and tangles in the brain of a deceased fifty-six-year-old demented patient, Auguste D. Each scientist at that gathering had made one or more historic discoveries in Alzheimer's disease research. Frankly, with all this new information, I was amazed to find myself swimming in a calming pool of scientific discovery and optimism.

Throughout the rest of 2007, with the encouragement and tutelage of the expert staff of the National Institute on Aging's Division of Neuroscience, under the guidance of Marcelle Morrison-Bogorad, PhD, and the Alzheimer's Association's highly respected chief medical and scientific officer, William Thies, PhD, our small team spoke with more than two hundred of the most active and cutting-edge American scientists and physicians working on this problem. We acknowledge with gratitude the spirit of generosity and enthusiasm of all those who helped educate us. Time and time again this research community reinforced our belief that now was the right time to inform the public about progress being made in Alzheimer's disease research. We learned about the research being conducted in multiple areas of basic science, drug development, and, to our surprise, lifestyle factors such as diet, exercise, and education that might mitigate the expression of the disease or delay its onset.

The scientists featured in the resulting documentary film, *Momentum in Science,* along with their discoveries and their present-day investigations, represent a near-complete portrait of the state of Alzheimer's disease research. Out of this film and all our research has come this book. Like the film, the book captures the excitement among scientists today, and explains their work in ways that we hope are easy to understand. We have placed the scientific discoveries in the broader context of the research field, highlighting what's most important and showing how it all fits together.

Part I of the book describes amazing breakthroughs in the basic science of Alzheimer's disease. Part II shows how new imaging technologies are making discoveries possible. Part III explores possible pathways to the disease, reflecting the new thinking that Alzheimer's disease is a disease of the whole body, not just the brain. Finally, Part IV looks at current work related to changing the disease process, including cutting-edge research on cognitive reserve and lifestyle factors, as well as the development of new drugs.

Working on the film and book has completely transformed the way I think about Alzheimer's disease. In the past, I had always assumed that my risk was very high because my father had the disease. In the course of this project, however, I learned that, while the general population has a 10 percent chance of developing Alzheimer's disease by age eighty-five, my father's illness increases my risk to 20 percent. Optimist that I am, I consider it that I have an 80 percent chance of not developing Alzheimer's. I find further comfort in the new term "susceptibility genes" to describe the role genetics plays in personal risk.

Late-onset Alzheimer's accounts for 97 percent of cases and is not *completely* determined by inheritance. Rather, a number of small genetic variations are believed to contribute to late-onset risk. Susceptibility, not inevitability. A vibrant worldwide race is under way to identify these susceptibility genes.

I have also been inspired by the prevailing view that the risk conferred by any single susceptibility gene is modified by the interaction of that gene with the environment. And, a considerable portion of what constitutes environment in this context is described as lifestyle factors. I encourage those who, like me, are worried about maintaining their cognition as they age, to pay particular attention to the compelling, and, to me, convincing research about lifestyle factors presented in Parts III and IV of this book. Scientific studies suggest that following a diet low in saturated fats and simple sugars, as well as maintaining normal levels of blood sugar, cholesterol, and blood pressure, may delay the onset of Alzheimer's disease or slow its progression. This same list of healthy lifestyle measures also minimizes one's chances of developing vascular dementia, the second leading cause of dementia. The book also presents exciting new research showing that aerobic exercise stimulates growth factors in the brain in the very areas first affected by Alzheimer's disease, in addition to its well-known cardiovascular benefits. These same growth factors, triggered by exercise, can reverse in animals the type of memory decline we all experience with normal aging.

If I had to reduce all the knowledge we have gleaned from the scientists profiled in *Momentum in Science* to one simple message, it would be that Alzheimer's disease is a disease of the entire body. Changes to any one system, such as the ability of insulin to deliver glucose to brain cells, may influence the metabolic pathways involved in Alzheimer's pathology. I'm fortunate that I don't have diabetes, but if I did, I'd be glad to know that there are ways to control such a problem. I am lucky that statins are available to control my cholesterol because, for me, diet and exercise are not effective enough on their own. I've been humbled and inspired to learn that my existence is a result of a remarkably complex, intricate, and delicately balanced system of metabolic pathways. Will my determination to keep my body, these systems, healthy have an impact on my old age? No one we met will guarantee this, but I do find comfort knowing that I am exerting control wherever I can.

In describing to friends and colleagues the experience of learning from these great minds and witnessing their research firsthand, I've often summarized my experience as: knowledge equals power. While I was by no means paralyzed by my anxiety, I had lived for too many years with a low-level dread that I was powerless over this situation—that my paternal genes could doom me to a decline into dementia. But now, after two years of immersion in Alzheimer's disease research, I feel a new sense of control over my future. I have lost my fear of Alzheimer's disease. I am proud that HBO and Public Affairs Books have collected this knowledge in *The Alzheimer's Project: Momentum in Science.* I hope that our work will inspire you not to feel powerless over how your whole body will age, but rather to stay informed, ask questions, and strive to keep your body and brain as healthy as possible.

JOHN HOFFMAN

ACKNOWLEDGMENTS

We are greatly indebted to the National Institute on Aging of the National Institutes of Health and to the Alzheimer's Association for all the support they have given us through the two years it took to produce *The Alzheimer's Project: Momentum in Science*. We are proud to have the NIA, the Alzheimer's Association, Fidelity Charitable Gift Fund, and the Geoffrey Beene Gives Back Alzheimer's Initiative as our copresenters.

We are grateful to the senior management of HBO, including our chairman and CEO, Bill Nelson; copresident Richard Plepler; documentary programming president, Sheila Nevins; and programming group president, Michael Lombardo, for continuing to foster an environment that allows projects like this to flourish. Every department at HBO has gone above and beyond in their efforts to extend the reach of *The Alzheimer's Project* to as large an audience as possible. This book would not have come to fruition without the tireless efforts of Jane Potenzo and Kati Madouros. We greatly appreciate their invaluable contributions.

Special thanks to all those who helped shape our thinking about Alzheimer's disease and guide us through the research landscape: Paul Aisen, MD; Dallas Anderson, PhD; Randy Bateman, MD; Thomas Beach, MD, PhD; David Bennett, MD; Neil Buckholtz, PhD; Randy Buckner, PhD; Vicky Cahan; Maria Carrillo, PhD; John Cirrito, PhD; Carl W. Cotman, PhD; Suzanne Craft, PhD; Charles DeCarli, MD; Steven T. DeKosky, MD; Anne Fagan, PhD; Niles Frantz; Dora Games, PhD; Angela Geiger; Alison Goate, DPhil; Todd Golde, MD; Robert C. Green, MD, MPH; John Hardy, PhD; Erin Heintz; Adrian Hobden, PhD; Richard J. Hodes, MD; David Holtzman, MD; Russell Katz, MD; William Klunk, MD, PhD; Eddie Koo, MD; Virginia Lee, PhD, MBA; Patricia Lynch; Chester Mathis, PhD; Richard Mayeux, MD; Marilyn M. Miller, PhD; Mark A. Mintun, MD; John C. Morris, MD; Marcelle Morrison-Bogorad, PhD; Lennart Mucke, MD; Suzana Petanceska, PhD; Ronald Petersen, MD, PhD; Creighton (Tony) Phelps, PhD; Joseph Rogers, PhD; Laurie Ryan, PhD; Marwan Sabbagh, MD; Gerard Schellenberg, PhD; Dale Schenk, PhD; Julie Schneider, MD; Mary Schwartz; Dennis J. Selkoe, MD; Sudha Seshadri, MD; Nina Silverberg, PhD; Scott A. Small, MD; Stephen Snyder, PhD; Larry Sparks, MD; Reisa Sperling, MD; William Thies, PhD; John Trojanowski, MD, PhD; Peggy Vaughn; Molly Wagster, PhD; Jennifer Watson; Howard Weiner, MD; MaryKate Wilson; Phil Wolf, MD; Wagner Zago, PhD; and Berislav Zlokovic, MD, PhD.

A special thanks to the dedicated team at Public Affairs: Peter Osnos, founder and editor-at-large; Susan Weinberg, publisher; Lindsay Jones, editor; and Melissa Raymond, managing editor.

THE SCIENTISTS

Paul S. Aisen, MD, professor of neurosciences at the University of California San Diego and director of the Alzheimer's Disease Cooperative Study, a consortium funded by the National Institute on Aging to develop assessment instruments and conduct clinical trials.

Randall J. Bateman, MD, assistant professor of neurology at the Washington University School of Medicine and clinical core leader in the Dominantly Inherited Alzheimer Network, a National Institute on Aging–funded study.

Thomas Beach, MD, PhD, head of the Civin Laboratory for Neuropathology and director of the Brain and Body Donation Program at Banner Sun Health Research Institute in Sun City, Arizona.

David A. Bennett, MD, director of the Rush Alzheimer's Disease Research Center at Rush University Medical Center in Chicago and principal investigator of the Religious Orders Study and the Rush Memory and Aging Project.

Randy L. Buckner, PhD, professor of psychology and neuroscience at Harvard University and an investigator with the Howard Hughes Medical Institute.

Carl W. Cotman, PhD, professor of neurology and director of the Alzheimer's Disease Research Center at the University of California Irvine.

Suzanne Craft, PhD, associate director of the Geriatric Research, Education, and Clinical Center of the VA Puget Sound and professor of psychiatry and behavioral sciences at the University of Washington School of Medicine.

Charles DeCarli, MD, professor of neurology and director of the University of California Davis Alzheimer's Disease Research Center.

Steven T. DeKosky, MD, vice president, dean, and James Carroll Flippin Professor of Medical Science of the Department of Neurology at the University of Virginia School of Medicine.

Alison Goate, DPhil, professor of genetics and neurology and associate director of the Alzheimer's Disease Research Center at Washington University School of Medicine and a co-investigator for the NIA's Alzheimer's Disease Genetics Consortium.

John Hardy, PhD, professor of neuroscience at the University College London Institute of Neurology.

Richard J. Hodes, MD, director of the National Institute on Aging, the National Institutes of Health, and the U.S. Department of Health and Human Services.

William E. Klunk, MD, PhD, professor of psychiatry and neurology and codirector of the Alzheimer Disease Research Center at the University of Pittsburgh.

Virginia M.-Y. Lee, PhD, MBA, John H. Ware 3rd Professor in Alzheimer's disease research in the Department of Pathology and Laboratory Medicine at University of Pennsylvania School of Medicine, director of the university's Center for Neurodegenerative Disease Research, and codirector of the Marian S. Ware Alzheimer Drug Discovery Program.

Chester A. Mathis, PhD, professor of radiology, pharmacology, and pharmaceutical sciences and director of the Positron Emission Tomography Facility at the University of Pittsburgh.

Richard Mayeux, MD, Sergievsky Professor of neurology, psychiatry, and epidemiology and codirector of the Taub Institute for Research on Alzheimer's Disease and the Aging Brain at Columbia University in New York; national director of the NIA Aging Family Study of Alzheimer's Disease.

John C. Morris, MD, Harvey A. and Dorismae Hacker Friedman Distinguished Professor of neurology and director of the Alzheimer's Disease Research Center Memory and Aging Project at Washington University School of Medicine.

Lennart Mucke, MD, director of the Gladstone Institute of Neurological Disease in San Francisco and professor of neuroscience at the University of California San Francisco.

Ronald C. Petersen, MD, PhD, Cora Kanow Professor of Alzheimer's Disease Research and director of the Mayo Alzheimer's Disease Research Center and the Mayo Clinic Study of Aging.

Joseph Rogers, PhD, founder and director of the Banner Sun Health Research Institute.

Gerard D. Schellenberg, PhD, professor in the Department of Pathology and Laboratory Medicine at the University of Pennsylvania and founder and head of the Alzheimer's Disease Genetics Consortium.

Dale B. Schenk, PhD, executive vice president and chief scientific officer for Elan Pharmaceuticals.

Dennis J. Selkoe, MD, Vincent and Stella Coates Professor of Neurologic Diseases at Harvard Medical School and codirector of the Center for Neurologic Diseases at Brigham and Women's Hospital.

Scott A. Small, MD, neurology researcher at Columbia University.

Reisa Sperling, MD, associate professor in neurology at Harvard Medical School, director of clinical research in the Memory Disorders Unit at Brigham and Women's Hospital, and director of the Neuroimaging Program at the Massachusetts Alzheimer's Disease Research Center at the Massachusetts General Hospital.

William Thies, PhD, chief medical and scientific officer of the Alzheimer's Association.

John Q. Trojanowski, MD, PhD, William Maul Measey-Truman G. Schnabel Jr., MD, Professor of Geriatric Medicine and Gerontology at the University of Pennsylvania School of Medicine.

Berislav V. Zlokovic, MD, PhD, dean's professor and director of the Center for Neurodegenerative and Vascular Brain Disorders and director of the Interdisciplinary Program in Dementia Research at the University of Rochester.

IMAGE CREDITS

Illustrations on pages ii, 3, 13, 14, 18, 32, 34—by Jannis Productions/courtesy of the National Institute on Aging

Images and photographs on the following pages:

vii, xi, xvii, 11, 25, 26, 44, 53, 91, 109, 119, 127, 128, 133, 143, 145, 147, 149, 150, 157—Katja Heinemann/HBO

1, 40, 41—provided by Dr. Lennart Mucke

8, 9, 15, 16—provided by Dr. Dennis Selkoe

29—provided by Dr. John Trojanowski and Dr. Virginia Lee

43—Jim Wehtje/Photodisc

57—provided by Dr. William Klunk/courtesy of Uppsala University PET Centre

65—courtesy of University of Pittsburgh PET Amyloid Imaging Group

78, top of 79—provided by Dr. Reisa Sperling

83—top image provided by Dr. Scott Small

85, 123—provided by Dr. Joseph Rogers/courtesy of *Neurobiology of Aging*

91—top photo provided by Dr. Alison Goate/courtesy of *Nature*

101—provided by Dr. Thomas Beach

106—provided by Dr. Berislav Zlokovic

117—provided by Dr. Suzanne Craft

129, 167—image provided by Wagner Zago at Elan Pharmaceuticals

160—courtesy of the Alzheimer's Association

All other images courtesy of HBO

I

HOW THE BRAIN CHANGES

Scientists have said that the human brain is the most complicated organ in the body—in fact, many claim that it is the single most complex natural or man-made entity on our planet. The mighty brain we carry in our heads processes billions of messages a minute, day and night, week after week, year after year, decade after decade. Its knowledge base expands and grows more complex with every new bit of information acquired, making informed decisions and taking creative leaps based on this new input, all the while retaining the older bits.

Tens of billions of nerve cells, called neurons, most smaller than a grain of sand, are compressed into an incredibly small space about the size of a cantaloupe. Each has a defined function, carrying out billions of distinct communications as we go through our day. At the same time, outside our awareness, the brain regulates breathing, heartbeat, digestion, sensory organs, excretion, and other functions. The brain is so important that even though it accounts for only 2 percent of our body weight, it receives 20 percent of our blood supply.

Yet we give little thought to our brain until we encounter a problem in our ability to think. If Alzheimer's disease (AD) develops, the brain slowly loses its ability to make and retrieve memories and process information. A friend's name that was once familiar now eludes us. Last week's Thanksgiving dinner draws a blank. A naval engineer who once performed algebra, calculus, and trigonometry can no longer balance his checkbook. A grandmother cannot recall her family's favorite cookie recipe and is not even safe in the kitchen anymore, as she forgets to shut off the oven. Bits and pieces of life are lost—a doctor's appointment, a child's birth date, the name of a flower, even a spouse's face. Eventually, even simple thinking skills are lost.

We don't yet have all the answers about what triggers the cascade of events that eventually leads to AD, or why some changes in memory and thinking skills that occur even in healthy aging become much more destructive in people who have the disease. But we have learned a lot about the major characteristics of the disease and the ways in which it develops over time. We also know that the processes in the brain that lead to the physical and behavioral changes in people with AD begin long before anyone is aware that a problem exists—ten to twenty years before significant memory loss occurs.

Part I will introduce several scientists whose pioneering research laid the foundation of our current knowledge about AD, and who continue to make important new findings. Their discoveries, and those of many other scientists devoted to AD research, have paved the way for recent advances in diagnosis and treatment.

The First Discovery

In 1906, the German psychiatrist Dr. Alois Alzheimer described the case of Auguste D., a woman of fifty-one who had been admitted to the hospital five years before her death with a series of symptoms that included problems with memory and comprehension, an inability to

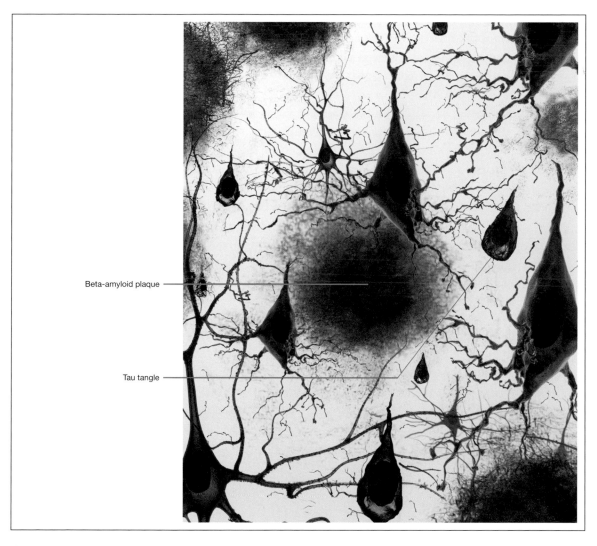

Beta-amyloid plaque

Tau tangle

This scientific drawing shows the damage caused by AD: beta-amyloid plaques, tau tangles, and the loss of connections between neurons.

speak, disorientation and hallucinations, and behavioral issues. After she died, Dr. Alzheimer performed an autopsy. Examining her brain tissue under a microscope, he found two unusual pathologies. One of these was a massive amount of sticky, insoluble proteins lodged in the spaces between nerve cells. Today these are called beta-amyloid plaques. The other was tangled bundles of protein threads within the neurons themselves, now called neurofibrillary tangles. Plaques and tangles are now considered the hallmarks of AD.

When Dr. Alzheimer made his seminal discovery, few took notice. At that time, the most common cause of dementia was syphilis.

In his day, he was much better known for his studies of this type of dementia than for the relatively infrequent Alzheimer's disease. Also, Alzheimer's disease was not as common then, because few people lived to seventy-five, the average age of onset. People only lived to forty-seven or forty-eight in 1900. (The top ten killers were infectious disease, like pneumonia, small pox, influenza, and venereal diseases.)

In 1910, the condition characterized by plaques, tangles, and accompanying symptoms was first called "Alzheimer's disease" by Dr. Alzheimer's supervisor at the Royal Psychiatric Clinic in Germany. However, for fifty years following Dr. Alzheimer's discoveries, knowledge about the disease grew slowly. Continuing improvements

Dementia

People often use "dementia" and "Alzheimer's disease" interchangeably, but the two words do not mean the same thing. Dementia describes a cluster of symptoms from a loss of cognitive skills—thinking, remembering, and reasoning—that is so severe the person has trouble carrying out daily activities.

Dementia usually is caused by a disease or condition. Sometimes it results from neurodegenerative diseases, like Alzheimer's disease or Parkinson's disease. In fact, Alzheimer's disease is the most common cause of dementia and today as many as five million Americans may have the disease. A stroke in the memory or language part of the brain also can create cognitive impairments that constitute dementia, but this dementia, a result of vascular disease, is referred to as vascular dementia. In other cases, dementia has a treatable cause. For example, the cumulative side effects of medications taken for other medical conditions can diminish the ability to remember and think. Depression, blood clots pressing on the brain, and metabolic imbalances also can lead to a dementia-like condition.

In the early stages of memory loss and other cognitive problems, it can be hard to distinguish between AD and other possible causes of dementia. That's one reason why many researchers are focusing so intently on the very early stages of AD. Not only do they want to understand what triggers and worsens the disease process, they want to develop sensitive, accurate diagnostic tools and tests. An early and accurate assessment of troubling signs and symptoms is crucial for encouraging people to get the treatment that matches their actual condition. Even though there are currently too few effective remedies, finding out early that troubling symptoms are caused by AD can help the person get into treatment early, before it is too late to intervene, and while current medications may have some chance of helping the person maintain cognitive function for a longer time. Early diagnosis also helps the person with AD and their family plan for the future and make the most of the time available to them.

in scientific instruments and methods allowed scientists to conduct more sophisticated studies of the biological structure of plaques and tangles. They began to recognize that the "Alzheimer's disease" defined as plaques and tangles occurring in the brains of relatively young adults were, in fact, the same structures they saw at autopsy in the brains of older people who had "senile dementia," the result of what was then called "hardening of the arteries."

The common assumption was that forgetfulness was a normal part of old age. Most people thought, "Uncle Fred is going through his second childhood," or "Grandma just can't remember where she puts things, but it's no big deal." During the 1960s, though, there was growing recognition that dementia was not, in fact, a normal part of aging but was often caused by a disease of the brain, Alzheimer's disease.

Since then, discoveries in Alzheimer's disease have come increasingly rapidly. We know now that, in most cases, symptoms of the disease emerge after age sixty-five; this is called late-onset AD. In a small number of cases, people develop the disease in their thirties, forties or fifties; this is called early-onset AD. Breakthroughs in the field of genetics have shown that early-onset cases run in families and are the result of particular genetic mutations. Late-onset AD probably results from a combination of genetic, environmental, and lifestyle factors. In both forms, the disease has the same pathology—the accumulation of beta-amyloid in plaques and neurofibrillary tangles that disrupt communication among neurons, ultimately leading to cell death.

What Happens in the Brain in Alzheimer's Disease?

One of the primary functions of neurons in the brain is to communicate with each other. One to two decades before symptoms of AD appear, communication begins to be disrupted. In a small region of the hippocampal formation, deep within the brain (called the entorhinal cortex), neurons begin to work less efficiently, probably because abnormal proteins begin to accumulate, forming neurofibrillary tangles. The damage then spreads to adjacent regions of the hippocampal formation, where, in addition to tangles, plaques are also formed. This brain region plays a major role in learning and is thought to be the brain's memory center, responsible for converting short-term memories into long-term memories. Long-term memories are then stored in other parts of the brain. Consider this conversion process as similar to clicking SAVE on a computer to store a paragraph in your computer's long-term memory. The brain absorbs information, holds it in short-term memory, and then converts short-term to long-term memory. This complex process depends on the ability of neurons to communicate with each other, and is disrupted by the onset and progression of Alzheimer's disease.

As tangles accumulate on the inside of neurons, and plaques accumulate on the outside of neurons, an increasing number of neurons become sick and die. Brain tissue in that area begins to shrink. Gradually, cell sickness and death spreads beyond the hippocampal formation. Over the course of years, this process overtakes much of the cerebral cortex—the gray matter, or outer shell of the brain—and it, too, degenerates. Nerve cells no longer communicate with each other and die. Fluid-filled spaces in the brain, called ventricles, enlarge as these other regions shrink, and the brain slowly loses its ability to create thoughts, experience emotion, or plan actions. Because the hippocampal formation is disrupted early, memory changes are among the first symptoms. As the disease progresses and other regions of the brain fall victim, more cognitive skills are affected and other symptoms appear. Eventually, people with AD are unable to carry out even simple tasks.

This book focuses on some of the leading scientists probing the secrets of Alzheimer's disease at the earliest phases of the disease process. It describes truly exciting work that is raising hopes for future diagnostic, monitoring, treatment, and even prevention strategies. To understand the potential impact of this work, it is important to first look at how Alzheimer's disease develops over time.

The Stages of Alzheimer's Disease

Though the time from diagnosis to death differs among people with Alzheimer's disease, the disease generally progresses through the same stages.

Dr. Ron Petersen was the first to define a condition called mild cognitive impairment (MCI) to describe early changes in memory. Dr. Petersen defined MCI as a condition in which a person has memory problems greater than expected for a person that age, but does not have the other cognitive or personality changes that typically accompany

AD. People with MCI are an important group for researchers to understand because about 80 percent of people with MCI characterized by memory loss go on to develop AD within seven years. (In contrast, only from 1 to 3 percent of people older than sixty-five with healthy cognitive abilities will develop AD in any given year.)

The definition and description of MCI has been a big advance because it provides a framework in which experienced clinicians, using sophisticated neuroimaging techniques and sensitive memory and cognitive tests, can monitor a person's cognitive changes over time. Being able to characterize and track cognitive changes is critical to determining whether a person has AD and when treatment may be most effective.

Over time, as the plaques and tangles continue to proliferate, an individual with MCI may progress to a clinical diagnosis of Alzheimer's disease. This stage is called mild, or early, Alzheimer's disease. More of the cerebral cortex will be affected, so memory loss will increase, and other cognitive abilities will diminish. An individual with mild AD may get lost in familiar places or fail to recognize his surroundings. He may take longer to accomplish the daily tasks of living like washing, dressing, and eating. He may have trouble handling money or paying bills or exercise poor judgment. Mood and personality changes can also occur; he may lose spontaneity or drive, or show increased anxiety or aggression. Although a person with mild AD may still seem healthy, it will be harder for him to make sense of his world. Although the individual and his family members and friends may have been aware of troubling changes for some time, AD is often diagnosed during this phase. The diagnosis often helps families make sense of their loved one's behaviors.

As Alzheimer's disease progresses and the damage spreads further in the brain, the person enters a stage referred to as moderate Alzheimer's disease. The brain continues to shrink and symptoms become more pronounced as the disease reaches the areas of the cerebral cortex that control language, reasoning, sensory processing, and conscious thought. A person with moderate AD may wander or become confused, anxious, or agitated, engaging in angry outbursts, tearfulness, irritability or restlessness. His attention span may shorten. He may have problems recognizing family and friends, and difficulty with language, reading, writing, and arithmetic, and with the logical organization of thoughts. He may be unable to learn new things and consequently be unable to cope with new situations. At this stage, a person with AD might also experience hallucinations and paranoid delusions, and lose impulse control, leading to things like inappropriate undressing or the use of vulgar language. It is helpful for caregivers to understand the disease and to be more prepared for these sorts of behaviors before they happen, and to know that it is the disease that is causing them.

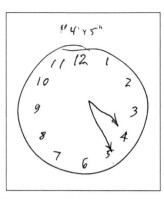

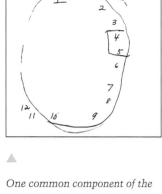

A person with moderate AD may be unable to carry out activities that require him to follow a sequence, like getting dressed or setting the table. Anger may mask anxiety and confusion. According to the National Institute on Aging, a person at the moderate stage of AD "may angrily refuse to take a bath or get dressed because he does not understand what his caregiver has asked him to do. If he does understand, he may not remember how to do it."

At the last stage of this illness, severe Alzheimer's disease, plaques and tangles are found throughout the brain. Most areas have shrunken further, leaving only a thin ribbon of gray matter and even larger fluid-filled ventricles. An individual at this final stage cannot communicate in any way except moaning and grunting. He doesn't recognize loved ones and is completely dependent on others for care. He may experience weight loss and difficulty swallowing, seizures, skin infections, lack of bladder and bowel control, and increased sleeping. If bedridden, he is likely to die from pneumonia as a result of having inhaled food or drink because of difficulty swallowing.

One common component of the cognitive exams used to help diagnose AD is referred to as "the clock test." As people experience cognitive decline, their ability to construct a clock accurately and have it indicate a specific time diminishes. Doctors can track the progress of the disease by asking patients to complete this task on repeat visits.

The Scientists of Part I

Scientists know that the major characteristics of AD in the brain are beta-amyloid plaques and neurofibrillary tangles. They also know how the disease progresses and the symptoms typical to each stage of the disease. Part I will give you an inside look at the work of several of the scientists who opened the doors to a deeper understanding of AD.

Chapters 1 and 2 highlight the scientists who have laid the foundation of our current understanding of beta-amyloid and tau, the two abnormal proteins that constitute plaques and tangles. Their work has major implications for future treatment and prevention strategies.

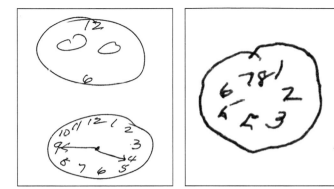

In Chapter 1, we will look at the role of beta-amyloid in the development of amyloid plaques. Dr. Dennis Selkoe has made breakthrough discoveries about beta-amyloid and why it is so toxic. We will also examine Dr. Randy Bateman's work. Since beta-amyloid itself is a normal part of our brain chemistry and healthy people produce and clear it out all the time, Dr. Bateman is studying why some people either produce too much of it or clear it less effectively.

In Chapter 2, we will follow the development of neurofibrillary tangles, the second hallmark of Alzheimer's disease, which the pioneering work of Dr. John Trojanowski and Dr. Virginia Lee has helped to reveal. Dr. Lennart Mucke has been conducting fascinating experiments into how the tau protein might damage cells.

Alzheimer's disease develops over many years, and by the time of diagnosis, the disease is often well advanced. Chapter 3 highlights the urgent work of scientists to understand the earliest stages of AD and to develop ways to identify people with memory problems who will go on to develop AD, and those who will not. Their work has major implications for future diagnosis, treatment, and prevention strategies. Dr. Ron Petersen will describe the diagnosis of mild cognitive impairment. This new understanding of the transitional stage from a healthy cognitive state to a disease state will eventually help primary practitioners diagnose and treat people who are likely to progress to AD. In Chapter 3, we also look at Dr. John Morris's new memory evaluation techniques, which may eventually become part of standard medical practice.

The excitement among these brilliant researchers is clear. Scientists today are moving closer to understanding how Alzheimer's disease changes the brain, the first step toward treatment and prevention.

1

UNDERSTANDING PLAQUES

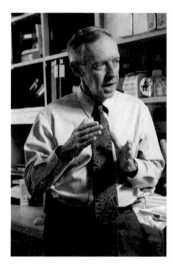

Striding through his lab at Brigham and Women's Hospital in Boston, **Dr. Dennis Selkoe,** a lean, intense man with piercing blue eyes, moves with a sense of mission. When he described to us what he believes is at the root of Alzheimer's disease, his excitement was palpable.

"For some three decades scientists around the world have been struggling with what causes Alzheimer's disease," he said. "How does it begin? How does it unfold? It has been a tough problem to address. But this is what we think is happening in certain parts of the person's brain." Dr. Selkoe explained that brain cells use chemically mediated electrical signaling to send messages to each other across a tiny gap called a synapse. This is how brain cells communicate with each other, and it makes possible all the conscious decisions and unconscious functions for which the human brain is responsible. A single transmission is like a tiny chemical signal traveling in the minute space between two cells. Trillions of these interactions happen every day.

In Alzheimer's disease, something goes terribly wrong. Slowly over time, the number of signals coming from certain neurons diminishes. "The synapse goes cold. It no longer transmits information properly. Eventually, the entire cell dies, and there is no more transmission. Eventually, this pattern occurs throughout the brain and is the centerpiece of Alzheimer's disease. At its core, the disease is a synaptic failure. When certain synapses are not working properly, we can't remember."

When synaptic transmission fails, the brain circuits that are needed to encode, or preserve, an experience in memory cannot do it, or can do it only imperfectly. "My patients will sometimes remember one thing about a Thanksgiving dinner a year ago, but are unable to recall other features. They lose the ability to encode new information they've heard or seen for the first time into a series of signals that make an imprint in the brain. When this slowly evolving process starts having a clinical impact, people not only can't put down new memories efficiently, but they also can't retrieve some memories from the memory bank. The problem isn't just with input; it's also with outflow— from something that was there at one time." Thus begins the slow, sad progression toward brain shrinkage and death.

The question of what causes neurons to stop communicating and die is complex. Recently, many scientists around the world have synthesized a hypothesis of how, in Dr. Selkoe's words, "Alzheimer's disease does its dirty work." He believes that although considerable bits of information are still lacking, enough is known about how the disease begins and causes trouble in the brain that scientists can now design and test ways to interrupt the process.

Dr. Selkoe has spent decades studying plaques and their major component, the protein fragment called a beta-amyloid peptide. His discoveries have contributed enormously to our understanding of the Alzheimer's disease process.

The Cutting of Amyloid Precursor Protein

In the mid-1980s in several laboratories around the world, beta-amyloid peptide was identified as the building block of plaques. Dr. Selkoe and his team contributed to this research, perhaps most importantly by developing the methods used in the preparation of contamination-free plaque cores. They soon found that beta-amyloid is produced by healthy cells throughout the body and throughout life, and can be easily detected in cultured cells (living cells that are grown in the laboratory for use in scientific studies). This finding inspired scientists around the world to focus on the formation of beta-amyloid and how it contributes to the development of Alzheimer's disease.

We have learned from genetic studies that beta-amyloid begins as a small part of amyloid precursor protein, or APP, a large protein thought to be important to the health of neurons. Like all proteins in the body, APP is constantly being generated and broken down. (Once they have served their purpose, all types of proteins are broken down and cleared away. This basic process is regulated by enzymes and other specialized "disposal" proteins.) As it is being made, the long, curly APP protein is tucked into the membrane of the neuron. The strand stretches from within the nerve cell, through the cell wall, to the outside of the cell.

At some point, for reasons still unknown, the segment of APP outside the cell is cut into fragments by enzymes. Dr. Selkoe refers to these enzymes as "molecular scissors."

Yet another major breakthrough occurred when scientists discovered that the cutting of APP can follow two very different pathways,

LEFT: *APP (purple) embedded in the cell membrane.*

RIGHT: *When alpha-secretase (green) cuts the APP molecule within the section that produces beta-amyloid, a harmless fragment is released. A second cut by gamma-secretase (turquoise) leaves the tail portion of APP in the cell; again, no toxic fragment is created.*

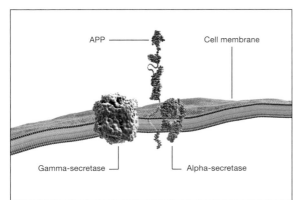

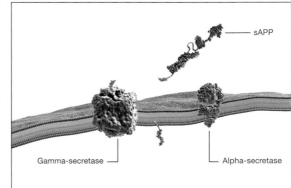

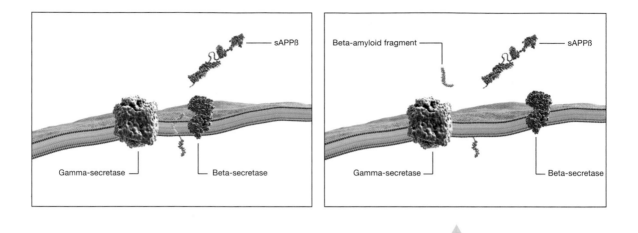

LEFT: *The beginning of a harmful sequence. Beta-secretase (magenta) cuts the APP molecule and releases a protein fragment called sAPPβ (purple).*

RIGHT: *Next, gamma-secretase (turquoise) cuts the fragment that is still tethered in the cell's membrane, releasing a small peptide: the toxic beta-amyloid (yellow).*

depending on which enzyme does the cutting, or cleaving, and where the cleavage occurs along the APP molecule. One path leads toward AD, while the other does not.

In the harmless pathway, an enzyme called alpha-secretase cuts the APP molecule correctly, and it can no longer become the harmful beta-amyloid peptide. This large fragment called sAPPα is released into the space outside the neuron, where it helps neurons grow and survive. In a later step on this harmless pathway, a second enzyme, gamma-secretase, cuts the part of APP still anchored within the nerve cell membrane. One of the two resulting fragments is also released to the outside of the cell, and the other fragment is released from the cell membrane but remains inside the cell, where it may enter the nucleus. No beta-amyloid is produced in this sequence.

In the harmful pathway, the enzyme beta-secretase cuts the APP molecule at one end of the portion that has the potential to become the toxic beta-amyloid. This releases a large fragment of APP called sAPPβ, whose role in the biology of the brain is unknown. Then an enzyme known as gamma-secretase cuts the remaining piece of APP molecule at the other end of what will become the beta-amyloid fragment. After it is cleaved at both ends, this fragment of APP, the beta-amyloid peptide, is released into the space outside the neuron.

Both of these cutting processes are entirely normal. They happen to all of us millions of times a day. Indeed, one of the crucial breakthroughs was the discovery that everyone makes beta-amyloid. "I'm pleased that ours was one of the labs to make that discovery in 1992," Dr. Selkoe said. "Before that, we thought beta-amyloid was only made through an obscure process of cell breakdown. But it's like forming cholesterol, which all of us make, too. It's a normal process."

Genetic investigations showed that families with early-onset AD had mutations in genes that code either for APP or for the two enzymes that cut the beta-amyloid molecule, and that this resulted in increased brain beta-amyloid and the development of the disease very early in life. These genetic discoveries led scientists to focus on beta-amyloid accumulation as a major cause of both early- and late-onset AD. The next question is how this normal process goes wrong.

From Peptides to Oligomers to Plaques

Put simply, people with Alzheimer's disease have too much beta-amyloid peptide in their brain. Whether some people make too much of it, or others clear too little of it, or both, is an open question. Nevertheless, the resulting imbalance is a central clue to understanding how a normal process can lead to a disease state.

In a high-powered microscopic view of a slice of the brain of a person with AD, one can see the classical abnormalities that the German psychiatrist Dr. Alois Alzheimer described: spherical deposits of amyloid plaques, surrounded by degenerating neurons and nerve endings. The plaques are made of many, many bits of the beta-amyloid peptide clumped together, along with other proteins, remnants of neurons, and other types of cells. If the creation of beta-amyloid is a normal process, how and why did these abnormal plaques develop?

This high-power microscopic view of brain tissue from a person with AD shows two beta-amyloid plaques surrounded by a halo of shrunken neurons, some of which clearly contain neurofibrillary tangles.

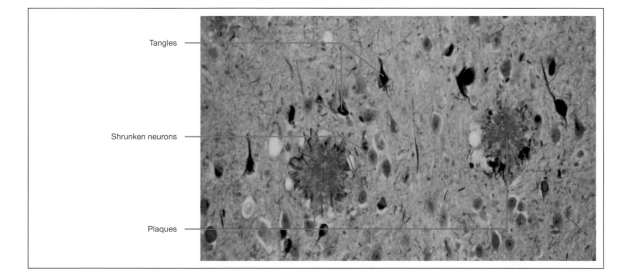

Tangles

Shrunken neurons

Plaques

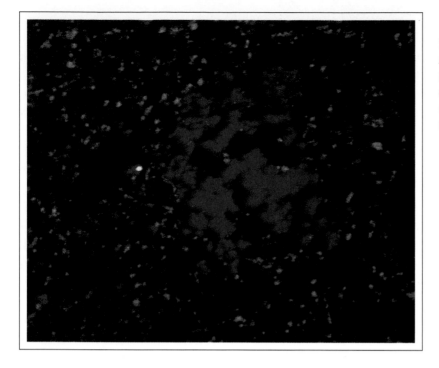

The red mass in this high-power microscopic picture is a typical beta-amyloid plaque in the brain of a person who died with AD; the green represents synapses in the surrounding tissue.

Dr. Selkoe believes that we now have the answer to this crucial question. If a single beta-amyloid peptide is present in the space between the nerve cells, it does not create a problem. But if the beta-amyloid cut from one APP molecule meets the beta-amyloid cut from another, they can stick together in twos, then threes, then fours, and so on. Clusters of a small number of beta-amyloid peptides are called oligomers, from the Greek word *oligos,* meaning "a few." They are rare in the brains of young people. But as we age, virtually everyone develops some beta-amyloid oligomers.

The brain has finely tuned mechanisms for clearing unwanted material like oligomers. It's likely that many oligomers are routinely and successfully cleared from the brain. In the brain of someone with AD, those that cannot be efficiently cleared begin to join with additional beta-amyloid peptides and oligomers, as well as other proteins and cellular material. As the process continues, the clumps of oligomers elongate into thin rope-like structures called amyloid fibrils that become increasingly difficult to clear away. Eventually, fibrils coalesce into the amyloid plaques that are characteristic of AD.

The Amyloid Cascade Hypothesis

One critical aspect of studying a complex disease like Alzheimer's disease is putting all the pieces of knowledge into a coherent and biologically plausible storyline that explains all the steps, from an initial potentially harmful event to the final, full-blown disease. In 1991, Dr. Selkoe formally proposed a chain of biological steps that lead to Alzheimer's disease in an article in the journal *Neuron*. Subsequently, he and other scientists refined and updated this concept as new knowledge accumulated. This "amyloid cascade hypothesis" posits that AD is a condition in which different kinds of genetic alterations, or non-genetic causes, can lead, directly or indirectly, to an overproduction of beta-amyloid or a decrease in its removal, in either case resulting in its excessive accumulation in the brain. The creation of beta-amyloid oligomers and plaques that results from this imbalance gradually leads to inflammation and other injury to brain cells, the formation of neurofibrillary tangles (the subject of the next chapter), and disruption of cellular communication. The end result is widespread loss of neurons and their synapses, causing memory decline and dementia.

Dr. Selkoe and many other AD researchers initially believed that it was the large, sticky amyloid plaques that were responsible for damaging the synapses and eventually leading to neuronal death. Recently, they have modified their thinking. Dr. Selkoe's current research has revised the hypothesis to focus on how tiny groupings of just two or three beta-amyloid peptides can enter the synapse, the miniscule space between two neurons over which the transmission of information occurs. If they get into the synapse, they short-circuit communication between adjacent neurons, damaging the synapse and eventually killing the neuron.

Even more surprisingly, Dr. Selkoe and other scientists have come to believe that the amyloid plaques themselves may not directly hurt neurons and may actually be protective in some way. "The amyloid plaque is large," Dr. Selkoe explained, "and I believe it cannot float into synapses and interfere directly with the electrical impulse. Larger is more protective, and smaller, especially very small, is not."

Nevertheless, the large amyloid plaques, composed of millions of beta-amyloid peptides and other cellular material, may not be entirely harmless. They may disrupt the pathways of neuronal extensions (axons and dendrites) by their mere presence. They may also shed beta-

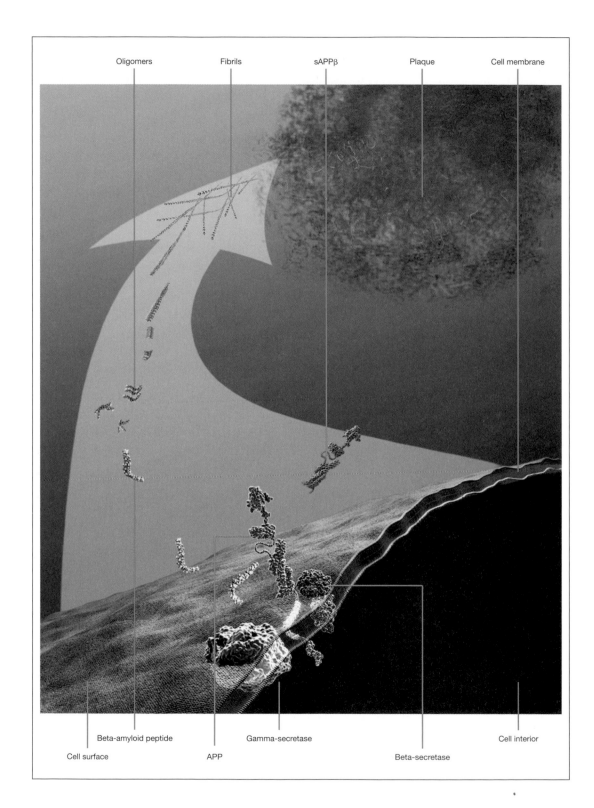

Oligomers Fibrils sAPPβ Plaque Cell membrane

Beta-amyloid peptide Gamma-secretase Cell interior

Cell surface APP Beta-secretase

amyloid oligomers and in doing so represent "a reservoir of badness," in Dr. Selkoe's words. "It's like saying a city has a large jail, and the jail is full. There are fewer criminals on the street, but eventually some of them can escape and cause trouble. Is it good to have amyloid plaques? In the short term, it is, because they keep the beta-amyloid peptides locked up. But there's a possibility of fragments getting out, where they can repopulate the brain's fluid space with beta-amyloid."

The final confirmation of the amyloid cascade hypothesis will come from controlled scientific studies of people who are treated with drugs designed to interfere with a step in the amyloid cascade. "The only way to prove this hypothesis and to make it truly self-evident is to show it in patients. We need to demonstrate that if we target the beta-amyloid, especially the oligomers, we can slow the progression of Alzheimer's disease."

An Unexpected Clue

Years ago, Dr. Selkoe and his colleagues examined the brain of a person who died with a large number of amyloid plaques in his brain. Remarkably, the slide was taken from a twelve-year-old.

"Many of us would be absolutely shocked to think that a twelve-year-old could have a buildup of beta-amyloid in the brain, forming millions of plaques, at an age when we simply can't imagine an Alzheimer-like disease process occurring. And yet this individual and other young people like him have this going on already."

This child had Down syndrome, which is also called trisomy 21. Through an accident in cell division, people with Down syndrome have an extra copy of chromosome number 21 in their cells. The gene that contains the information necessary to make the APP protein is located on chromosome 21, providing an enormously powerful clue. "When this was announced in 1986, it gave me an enormous sense of excitement," Dr. Selkoe told us. "Now we understood why Down syndrome automatically produces a highly premature form of Alzheimer's disease." Because people with Down syndrome have an extra copy of the APP gene, these individuals always have too much APP, and as this large protein is normally cut into pieces, they produce too much beta-amyloid, beginning before birth and continuing throughout life.

"We can measure the beta-amyloid peptide in the bloodstream shortly after a person with Down syndrome is born, and we know that there's too much. Eventually that beta-amyloid will build up, becoming observable under a microscope by the early teens. All people with Down syndrome, if they survive into their thirties or forties or beyond, have a brain picture that looks like full-blown Alzheimer's disease."

Beta-Amyloid in the Lab

Like many other investigators in this field, Dr. Selkoe's team uses mice because the biochemistry of synaptic function is essentially the same in mice and humans and, in fact, across all mammals. The transmitter molecules that spread a "message" from one nerve cell to another across a synapse are identical, and the genes and proteins that regulate neuron-to-neuron messaging seem virtually indistinguishable. In one test, Dr. Selkoe and his team floated large amyloid plaques isolated from the brains of people who had died of AD onto slices of normal adult mouse brain tissue. They found that the plaques themselves did not interfere with the electrical activity in the tissue, supporting the concept that the plaques were less dangerous than originally thought. They then succeeded in isolating oligomers of beta-amyloid peptides from the same brains of people with AD, even extracting them out of the amyloid plaques, to try to pinpoint which type of beta-amyloid was causing the trouble. They collected the gray matter from the cortex—a brain area markedly affected by AD plaques and tangles—and homogenized it (literally using a blender to create a fluid from the tissue). Then, in a centrifuge that spun at 150,000 times the force of gravity, they separated the insol-

Dr. Dennis Selkoe is studying whether small groupings of beta-amyloid—the types of oligomers called dimers and trimers—might be the culprits in the beta-amyloid cascade hypothesis, rather than larger plaques.

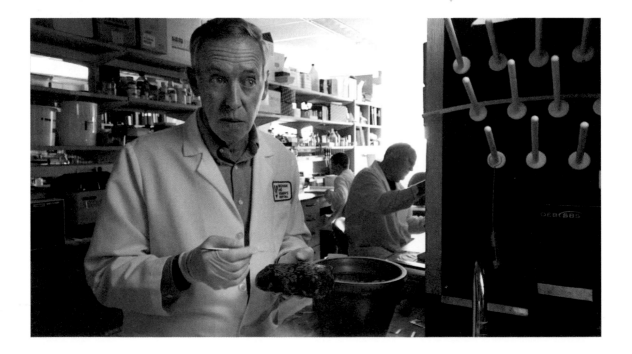

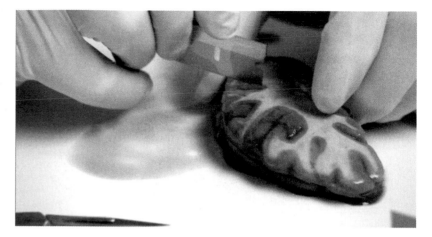

Researchers must isolate the gray matter of the brain, which contains greater concentrations of the beta-amyloid dimers and trimers than the white matter, in order to determine the toxicity of the oligomers.

uble amyloid plaques from a clear liquid, which rose to the top. Within the liquid they detected the small oligomers of beta-amyloid peptide. They then separated different sized oligomers as well as single peptides (called monomers). They bathed slices of mouse hippocampal formation with these various preparations.

The team learned that a single peptide caused no trouble; the electrical activity in the slice was normal. But a clump of two or three peptides, oligomers called dimers and trimers, dramatically impaired the electrical activity—just the type of response that would be expected if the "machinery" necessary for laying down new memories was impaired. This was an exciting finding. Using tissue preparations taken from the same region of the brain of a healthy older person, Dr. Selkoe's team showed that the number of synaptic transmissions remained high in the presence of the normal brain extract.

In a related series of experiments, Dr. Selkoe and his colleagues Dr. Dominic Walsh and Dr. Ciaran Regan, both at University College Dublin, wondered whether injecting beta-amyloid material from the brain of a person with AD into a healthy adult rat's brain would interfere with the rat's memory. To test this question, the team trained rats to do something they don't normally do.

Normal rats prefer the dark. The scientists devised a "rat apartment" with one well-lit chamber and one darkened one, with a door in between. They trained rats not to follow their natural instincts but to stay in the lighted chamber.

Then they introduced beta-amyloid oligomers isolated from the brain of a person with AD into a rat's brain to see if it would impair the rat's memory for this learned behavior. The results were dramatic.

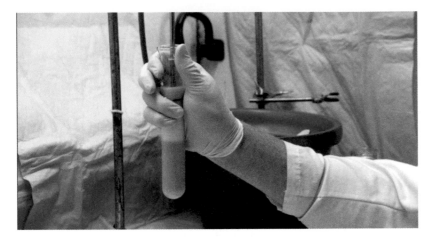

Once the scientists have isolated the gray matter, they purify it with this motor-driven tissue homogenizer to separate the beta-amyloid dimers and trimers from the rest of the gray matter.

When the researchers put miniscule amounts into the rat's brain, it quickly forgot it had learned not to enter the dark chamber and scampered right back into it. "The rat could no longer remember that learned behavior."

Working on a different set of rats, Dr. Selkoe's team then took this one step further and mixed the beta-amyloid material from the human brain with an antibody that binds to beta-amyloid, removing it from the fluid sample. When they put this beta amyloid-free fluid into the rat's brain, it remembered that it wasn't supposed to go into the dark chamber. "We were able to take material—specifically, beta-amyloid oligomers—from the human brain and show that it impairs memory in a healthy adult animal," Dr. Selkoe explained. "We isolated something that has potent activity on synapses, causing them to work improperly. That's what the field has been trying to achieve in many different experiments, in many different ways."

Controversy and Hope

New ideas like the amyloid cascade hypothesis are always controversial in science. As convincing as the theory and experiments of Dr. Selkoe and other scientists seem, they have not been universally accepted.

"There are some serious, legitimate criticisms," Dr. Selkoe told us. "Perhaps the most common one is that full-blown amyloid plaques—and therefore also oligomers and different forms of beta-amyloid—are present in elderly people who are doing fine. When they die, we see they had this amyloid, but still they had been performing quite well, which suggests to some people that beta-amyloid is not causing Alzheimer's disease."

This is a concern that Dr. Selkoe feels he can address. One possibility, he says, is that the amyloid plaques found in apparently well people may be protective, and that there may not be enough free-floating oligomers of beta-amyloid peptide to cause noticeable memory impairment. He suggests another possibility. "We know from studying many other diseases that people have managed to deal with a nasty disease process and show almost no external effects. For example, some people have bad atherosclerosis, yet never have a twinge of angina or a heart attack. I know people who died at eighty-five, ninety, ninety-five with so much atherosclerosis I can't believe they never had a heart problem. Even though a person shows no symptoms, does anyone conclude that regulating cholesterol and keeping atherosclerotic plaques from developing and preventing inflammation isn't a good treatment for preventing heart attack and stroke?" Correspondingly, although amyloid plaques may not themselves have a debilitating effect in all people, their excess presence, like cholesterol buildup, is not desirable.

Sometimes people who appear to be developing AD die of other causes before they have their first symptoms of forgetfulness. A chronic disease may have a very long pre-clinical phase before symptoms become evident. "We know from studying people who had a gene for early-onset AD, but died first of other causes, that plaque buildup may begin ten or twenty years beforehand. When we look at their brains under the microscope, we can see signs of Alzheimer's disease as long as twenty years before we expected the person would have become forgetful. In fact, upon autopsy, their brains sometimes look almost indistinguishable from people with bona fide AD. So I think the concern about amyloid plaques in apparently healthy people can be put to rest."

Another objection has to do with the second major hallmark of AD—tangles of tau protein, the subject of the next chapter. Some research papers suggest that if you look carefully for tangles, they can be found before there's any amyloid plaque in the brain. Dr. Selkoe has two answers. One is that most of those studies simply asked the question, "How and when do tangles appear in the aging human population?" Brains that came to autopsy at forty-five and fifty had a few tangles but no plaques. But no one knows whether those people, had they lived on, would have developed Alzheimer's disease later. Second, tangles, which are less specific than beta-amyloid plaques, appear in a dozen or more human diseases. "We can't say everyone who has tangles before plaques would have developed Alzheimer's. They may have developed another tangle disease. In fact, there are almost no examples of a terrible tangle buildup producing a secondary amyloid buildup. But the reverse is absolutely true. All the genetic mutations that we know to cause Alzheimer's disease start with beta-amyloid buildup and then lead to tau tangles."

Objections to the amyloid cascade hypothesis remind Dr. Selkoe of what the German philosopher Schopenhauer wrote two hundred years ago: All truth passes through three states. First, it is ridiculed. Second, it is violently opposed. Finally, it is accepted as being self-evident. "I'd like to think that will be the case for the hypothesis my colleagues and I have been working on. We're not quite there. I think we have enough information now that, although there are still missing links, we believe this hypothesis is worthy of vigorous pursuit."

Dr. Selkoe reflected on his long career. "When you pick a career and you work hard, if you're lucky you have about forty years or so to understand the field and make progress," he told us. "I entered this sometimes problematic but now increasingly promising area of what I call 'Alzheimerology' when I was young and when many techniques were about to emerge. Protein biology, which is what I've mostly worked in, has evolved in the last three decades right in front of my eyes.

"We can conduct our experiments in a much more sophisticated way now than when I was doing all my own experiments at the bench in the 1970s and 1980s. I've seen an explosion of interest in sophisticated methods in molecular biology and protein chemistry."

There has been so much progress in the field that it is attracting scientists from other disciplines who once would never have thought to work on AD because the research was messy and imperfect in the early days. "The brain was a black box for a long time. Now scientists view neuroscience as a very promising area for the near and distant future: as a way to understand what makes us human, understand the mind-brain relationship, understand prejudice, understand depression, understand shyness, understand what makes one personality attractive and another not. Those are things we're going to figure out.

"My great hope is that we will see a steady decline in the severity of Alzheimer's, that we will push back its onset, that we will shorten the time people suffer this terrible decline of their most human qualities. In fact, we now have treatments in hand and already have clinical trial results that suggest we're on the right track. We're not certain that we're one hundred percent correct. But so many of us in the field feel we're close enough that we can really start intervening."

A Thirty-Six-Hour Amyloid Test

Building on Dr. Selkoe's work, **Dr. Randy Bateman,** a neurologist at Washington University in St. Louis, has developed a new technique to measure the ebb and flow of beta-amyloid in the central nervous systems of people with and without Alzheimer's disease. Over the past few years, discoveries in his lab have shown that healthy young people make and clear beta-amyloid all the time.

Dr. Bateman is conducting research into some of the earliest changes in AD. He's focusing on changes in beta-amyloid in cerebrospinal fluid, the fluid found in and around the brain and spinal cord. This fluid cushions these organs and provides nutrients. "We already know that beta-amyloid exists in cerebrospinal fluid and that plaques are being deposited years before someone is diagnosed with the disease. Our study is attempting to look at what changes occur before that stage. We want to measure the changes in production or clearance of beta-amyloid so that we know what to look for even before the disease is diagnosed."

Dr. Bateman conducted preliminary studies with young healthy people, and followed up these studies with research in older individuals who have AD and those who don't.

Samples of cerebrospinal fluid are collected through a thirty-six-hour-long spinal tap.

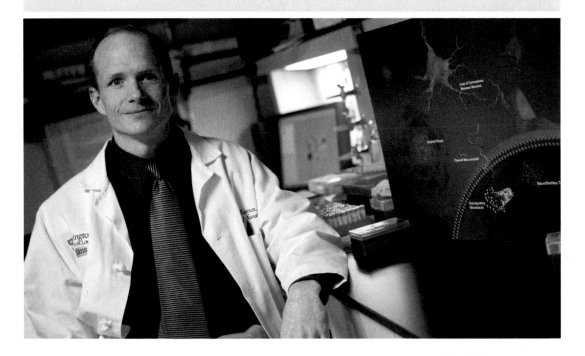

This may sound painful, but the research volunteers are comfortable during the procedure. A spinal catheter in their backs collects cerebrospinal fluid once an hour. "A single measurement would be like a still picture, a snapshot," Dr. Bateman explained to us, "It would give us a sense of the status of amyloid at that point in time, but we wouldn't know how it is changing. The thirty-six-hour study is like a movie. We're actually watching how beta-amyloid is being produced in the living brain, its rate of production, and how quickly it's being cleared away."

Proteins created in the body are made from building blocks called amino acids. The team infuses the study participants with an amino acid that has been labeled with carbon atoms that are a little heavier than normal carbon atoms. These amino acids exist normally in all of us; the only difference is the extra weight. Once this labeled amino acid gets into the bloodstream it is carried throughout the body and into the brain.

Proteins made in the brain after the infusion may incorporate one of these labeled amino acids into their structure. "As these newly made proteins are tagged with the heavy carbon atom, we can measure them. Over the test period, we can measure how quickly those newly generated beta-amyloid proteins are made and how quickly the body clears them away."

_____

Preparing a research volunteer for the insertion of a spinal catheter, which will measure the ebb and flow of beta-amyloid in his cerebrospinal fluid over thirty-six hours.

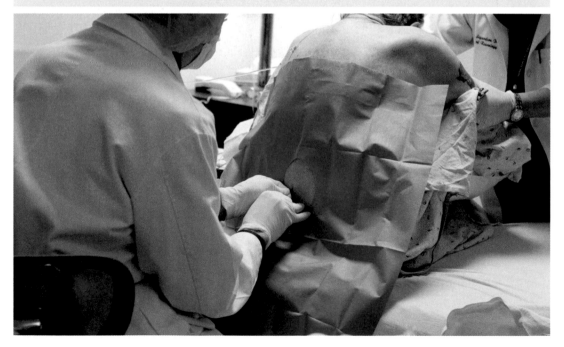

From the studies he has conducted in young healthy people, Dr. Bateman was able to demonstrate that beta-amyloid is produced very rapidly in our brains every day, and is also cleared away rapidly. It is a dynamic process. In fact, Dr. Bateman told us that young people make 8 percent of their beta-amyloid each hour, but they also eliminate it at the same rate. "In eight or nine hours, half the beta-amyloid in their brains will have been made and cleared away as normal functioning of the neurons."

Dr. Bateman also found that levels of beta-amyloid rose and fell dramatically during the day—sometimes by two- or threefold. In order to understand what caused the fluctuations, the research team recently added new components to this study.

"As we monitor beta-amyloid production," Dr. Bateman explained, "we now also measure the brain waves of our participants using an EEG (electroencephalogram). In addition, we videotape our research volunteers throughout the entire study period in time-lapse video. Just as the beta-amyloid levels are dynamic, a person's activities and brain functions change. Activities such as waking and sleep states, talking on the telephone, watching TV, and doing crossword puzzles alter brain activity. We are continuing to look for connections between their behaviors and those changing levels."

Dr. Bateman's colleague at Washington University, Dr. John Cirrito, has shown that when neurons communicate with each other, they produce beta-amyloid. This suggested to Bateman that fluctuating beta-amyloid levels may correlate with activity, behavior, or brain wave states, as measured by the EEG. Does working on a computer or talking on the phone always cause an increase in beta-amyloid? Does being in deep sleep decrease it? "Our hypothesis is that certain activities will cause it to go up and other activities will cause it to go down." Someday, this may lead to recommendations on activities to avoid or increase in order to affect APP metabolism, which in turn affects beta-amyloid production.

Dr. Bateman's research has implications for drug development, too. Because, like Dr. Dennis Selkoe, he believes that too much beta-amyloid causes the problems associated with AD, one possible treatment would be to reduce its production by blocking one of the two enzymes that cut APP in the process that leads to beta-amyloid. Drugs called beta-secretase inhibitors and gamma-secretase inhibitors have been developed to do just that. "It used to be challenging to show whether such a drug was effective in people with Alzheimer's disease, because it was difficult to measure the amount of beta-amyloid in the brain. The method we've developed to measure its production and clearance can now be applied to drug trials." This method has now been used in a gamma-secretase inhibitor currently in clinical trials.

The bottom line for Dr. Bateman: "Any way we can lower the level of beta-amyloid may be beneficial."

2

UNTANGLING TAU

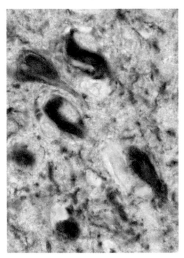

While much study has revolved around beta-amyloid plaques, for many years the role of neurofibrillary tangles, the other defining pathology of Alzheimer's disease, received much less attention. These tangles consist of abnormal bundles of a protein named tau, which exists within the neurons themselves (see the dark brown clusters in the image to the left). Scientists tended to focus on beta-amyloid because it was relatively specific to Alzheimer's disease and because it seemed to play a role in the genetics of early-onset AD. Less attention was directed to neurofibrillary tangles, possibly because they were present in other illnesses and were not caused by mutations in the tau protein. Most believed that the Alzheimer's disease–specific drug target to go after was beta-amyloid.

In recent years, however, tau research has generated new interest. One reason was the linking of tau and neurofibrillary tangles to several other neurodegenerative diseases. Significantly, scientists recently discovered multiple mutations in the tau gene that are responsible for a type of dementia caused called frontotemporal dementia. That type of dementia is the second most common cause of dementia after Alzheimer's disease in people under sixty years old.

Growing interest in tau and neurofibrillary tangles, the Alzheimer's disease brain pathology formed by abnormal tau proteins, is also the result of several decades of groundbreaking work by many scientists, including the ones in this chapter. **Dr. John Trojanowski** and **Dr. Virginia Lee,** a married couple, are codirectors of the Center for Neurodegenerative Disease Research at the University of Pennsylvania. Dr. Trojanowski is a pathologist, and Dr. Lee, a former classical pianist from China, is a biochemist. Their collaboration over the past two decades provided much of the foundation of our current knowledge about tau and tangles. Now they are applying that knowledge

Dr. John Trojanowski

▼

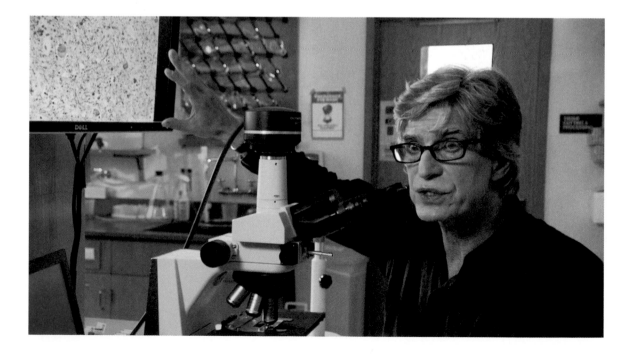

in the search for potential tau-related drug therapies. As always, the identification of each new step in the disease process provides the potential for a new drug target.

Later, we will meet Dr. Lennart Mucke, who has devoted his career to studying the Alzheimer's disease process from seemingly every angle. A fortuitous finding led him to investigate a new and provocative aspect of tau biology.

How Neurons Work

To understand tau and neurofibrillary tangles, it is necessary to know about the basic structure and function of a nerve cell. Most cells in the body are formed, live for a period of time, and die; new cells are constantly being generated to replace the ones that die. Unlike these cells, most neurons, which are formed in the developing embryo or fetus and shortly after birth, can live for up to one hundred years or longer. They cannot be replaced, so to remain healthy, neurons must continually maintain and repair themselves.

The human brain has billions of neurons. Each has a cell body that contains the cell's nucleus. The nucleus contains DNA, which

Dr. Virginia Lee
▼

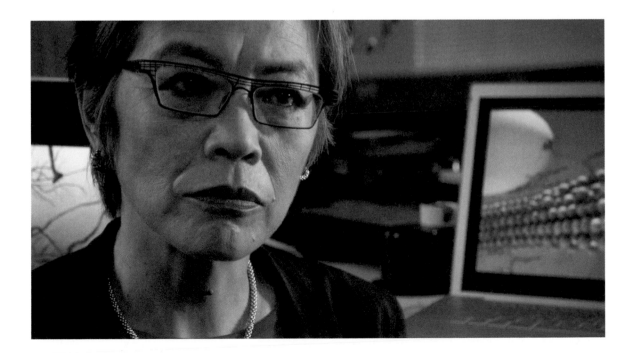

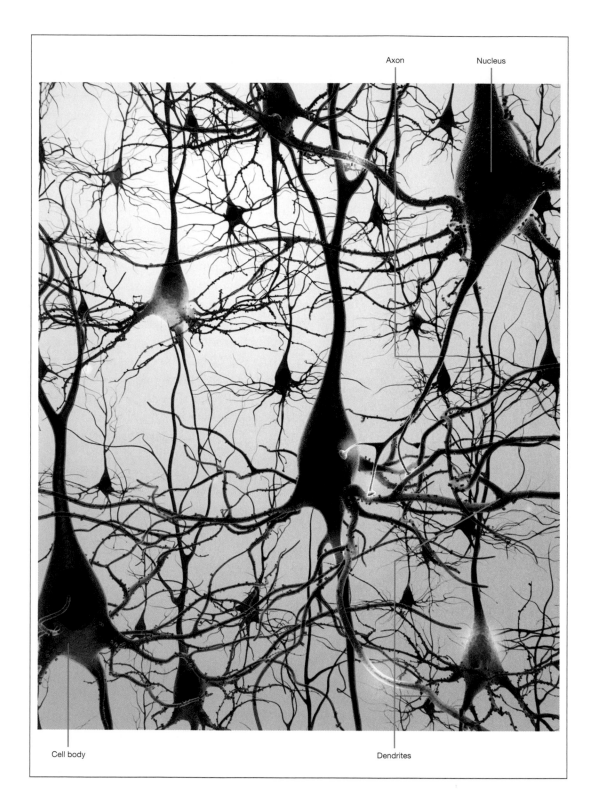

Axon

Nucleus

Cell body

Dendrites

controls much of the cell's activities. The nucleus is surrounded by the cytoplasm, which contains other structures, called organelles, with specific roles—such as the mitochondria, which produce the energy cells need to do their work. Neurons also have other structures, called axons and dendrites, that allow them to carry out their primary job of communicating with each other. An axon, which is much thinner than a human hair, extends out from the cell body. Axons transmit electrochemical messages to neighboring neurons by interacting with other neurons' dendrites, which carry signals to the next neuron, thereby conveying a message (like reading and understanding the words on this page) or producing an action (like turning this page to continue reading). The messages are transmitted across a gap called the synapse. Millions of neurons are communicating at any one time through their axons and dendrites.

When a message needs to be sent ("I feel pain! I just stubbed my toe!"), a nerve impulse is generated near the neuron's cell body. The impulse travels down the axon to its end, where a chemical messenger called a neurotransmitter is released. The neurotransmitter crosses the synapse to a specific receptor site on the next cell's dendrite. There, it fits into its receptor like a key in a lock to complete the communication. Depending on the signal it receives, the neighboring neuron either will intercept the new message and not pass it on, or will send the message to other parts of the brain. This communication happens instantaneously, so that within a split second of stubbing a toe, a person yells, "Ouch!" At any one time, millions of these signals are traversing the circuits and networks of the brain, sending, receiving, and processing enormous volumes of information, and directing other parts of the body how to react to stimuli.

Healthy neurons are supported by microtubules, or parallel tubular structures that allow movement of molecules up and down the axon and dendrites. Think of these as train tracks inside the axons and dendrites. This is where the protein tau comes into play: It holds the microtubules together like ties on train tracks and stabilizes them.

When Tau Becomes Abnormal

Dr. Trojanowski and Dr. Lee laid the groundwork for tau researchers by discovering that the tangles seen inside the neurons of people who died of Alzheimer's disease are composed of an abnormal form of the

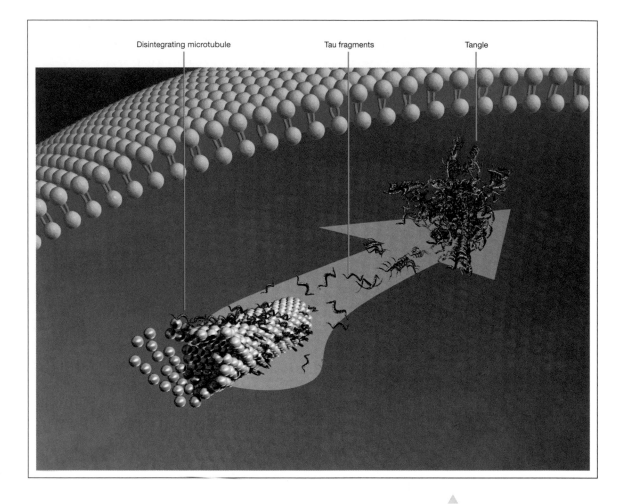

Disintegrating microtubule   Tau fragments   Tangle

Healthy neurons are supported in part by microtubules, but, in AD, tau detaches from the microtubules, causing the neuron's internal transport network to collapse.

tau protein. They also discovered the way in which tau becomes abnormal.

When Dr. Trojanowski and Dr. Lee started looking for the building blocks of neurofibrillary tangles the late 1980s, the composition of tangles was still not understood. "We began with brain tissue from people who died of Alzheimer's disease," Dr. Lee told us. "We isolated the tangles from the brain and were able to purify the protein to homogeneity," so that only the component of the tangles remained. "We obtained a protein sequence, the chemical identifier or bar code of the tau protein."

After years of meticulous biochemical experiments, they demonstrated what was wrong with the abnormal tau threads in the tangles. Tau in its normal state contains a limited number of phosphate mol-

ecules, but in the case of Alzheimer's disease they found an abnor-
mally large number of phosphate molecules attached to the tau, a situation described as hyperphosphorylation. These extra phosphate
molecules somehow cause the tau to detach from the microtubules,
disrupting the effectiveness of axonal transport. The microtubules lose
their structural support and collapse—similar to the way train
tracks buckle and fall apart with the loss of cross ties—resulting in
many "train wrecks" in the brain. The neuron's internal transport network collapses, damaging the axons and dendrites, leading to the cell's
inability to communicate with other neurons. The so-called "train
wrecks" become toxic dumps that accumulate and cause collateral
damage to the brain, while the threads of tau begin to form structures
called paired helical filaments, which join with other threads of tau,
ultimately creating neurofibrillary tangles. Eventually the cell dies.

"Identifying abnormal tau as this building block was equivalent
to identifying the virus that causes AIDS or polio," said Dr. Trojanowski. "It's the springboard from which diagnosis and eventually
therapeutic intervention will flow." Their work allowed investigators
to branch into many new scientific directions in their research on
Alzheimer's disease.

Misfolded Proteins

Having discovered the molecular building block of tau tangles, Dr.
Trojanowski and Dr. Lee began to ask some different questions about
the relationship of tau to Alzheimer's disease. They wanted to know
when in the disease process these changes in tau occurred, and how
the tangles might be responsible for the damage to brain tissue seen
in Alzheimer's disease.

When any protein in the body is formed, it is not a straight, thread-
like sequence; rather, it "folds" into a unique three-dimensional shape
that helps it perform its task. This crucial process can go wrong for
various reasons, and does so more frequently in aging cells. The protein can fold into an abnormal shape. Dr. Trojanowski explained the
consequences of misfolding. "Proteins are like this piece of paper,"
he told us, holding up a meeting agenda. "But if those proteins are
crumpled or misfolded, they lose functionality. When I crumple this
piece of paper, I can't read it. The information is here, but it's no longer
accessible to me because it has an abnormal configuration." If this

happens repeatedly, the buildup of this nonfunctioning misfolded protein can become toxic.

Dr. Trojanowski and Dr. Lee knew that in Alzheimer's disease both the beta-amyloid protein and the tau protein were misfolding. They also knew that other labs were working on other neurodegenerative diseases that also featured misfolded proteins. For example, Huntington's disease, Parkinson's disease, amyotrophic lateral sclerosis (ALS, also known as Lou Gehrig's disease), Lewy body disease, frontotemporal dementia, prion diseases, Creutzfeldt-Jacob disease ("mad cow" disease), and others all have this same pathologic hallmark: misfolded proteins. Many of these conditions have symptoms similar to Alzheimer's disease, including memory loss, movement problems, and sleep-wake disorders. Perhaps, reasoned Dr. Trojanowski and Dr. Lee, further investigations into misfolding could not only reveal some clues about the development of Alzheimer's disease but also provide insight into these other diseases.

Fortunately, cells usually repair or degrade misfolded proteins. "Natural mechanisms offset protein misfolding, which happens all the time," said Dr. Trojanowski. "The molecules that do this are called chaperones. They have the ability to repair misfolded proteins so that they regain their function, much like I can read my wrinkled agenda once I smooth it out." In addition, other molecules in the nerve cell, called lysosomes and proteasomes, act like trash compactors to dispose of misfolded proteins.

If too many misfolded proteins are formed as part of age-related changes, the body's repair and clearance process can be overwhelmed. This may happen when tau tangles begin to accumulate. "The trash compactor gets stuffed up," Dr. Trojanowski theorized, "and can't accept any more trash." Then the excess spills over and accumulates throughout the nerve cell, becoming toxic. "The accumulation of brain trash impedes the normal traffic inside the cell by putting up roadblocks. Soon, misfolded proteins begin sticking to other misfolded proteins to form insoluble aggregates."

The aggregates build up, obstruct the movement of neurotransmitters down the axon to the synapse, and disrupt the ability of the cell to carry out its normal activities. Eventually the cell is so damaged that it dies.

Research into misfolded proteins in age-related neurodegenerative diseases may lead to therapies. Dr. Trojanowski believes, "it's reasonable to be optimistic about learning lessons from Alzheimer's disease and translating them into insights that help us understand therapeutics for Parkinson's disease or amyotrophic lateral sclerosis."

Toward Reducing Tangle Formation

Dr. Trojanowski and Dr. Lee are currently working on the next step: reducing the formation of tangles. One theory they are now exploring involves minimizing the hyperphosphorylation of the tau protein. Preventing too many phosphate molecules from attaching to tau would help tau bind better to microtubules, helping them perform their normal function.

In 1995, Dr. Lee and a colleague at the University of Pennsylvania discovered that lithium chloride (a drug used to treat bipolar disorder) can inhibit an enzyme involved in the hyperphosphorylation of tau. Eight years later, in 2003, Dr. Lee showed that lithium could also inhibit beta-amyloid peptide production.

As Dr. Trojanowski explained, however, devising potential drug treatment strategies is not simple. Much research attention has been directed toward drug therapies that eliminate or block beta-amyloid in the brains of people with Alzheimer's disease. However, blocking plaque formation in people with Alzheimer's disease, even reversing it in people at an early stage of the disease, may not restore their memory function or stop further degradation of their memories because the tau tangles would still be present. By the time a person with Alzheimer's disease experiences memory loss, the buildup of beta-amyloid in his brain has somehow triggered the accumulation of tau tangles, which may prove to be the more disruptive pathology to cell communication.

"If you eliminate plaques, you might convert a person with Alzheimer's disease into one with a tau neurodegenerative disease in which he would still experience cognitive and motor impairments and other symptoms of neurodegeneration. It would be very troubling ten years from now if we do eliminate plaques and still find that we have not cured the disease. Although therapeutics that work by preventing plaque formation could prevent the whole disease cascade if they are given before the disease begins, once the disease is in process, tangles will have to be targeted as well."

Dr. Lee added, "If plaques do come first, it may be possible to identify the stage in the disease in which, if you can eliminate plaques, then tangles won't develop. But once people show symptoms, most likely they already have both plaques and tangles in the brain. By that point, it would be too late to target just one and not both."

Currently, Dr. Trojanowski and Dr. Lee are using an innovative new technology to search for potentially useful tau-targeted drug compounds. They are using a robot to screen hundreds of thousands of molecules. The robot allows them to perform a huge volume of screenings that would otherwise require thousands of hours and hundreds of people. Recently, they screened nearly three hundred thousand compounds in a few days. Once researchers have identified a compound that inhibits the formation of tau tangles, the next step is to take it to a cell model to determine whether it can do what it did in a test tube in the context of a whole cell.

The next step will be to test the same compound in an animal model of Alzheimer's disease. One of the biggest early barriers to answering the tau question was that researchers didn't have a good animal model to work with, since humans are the only known species to develop a dementia caused by tau tangles. Recently, scientists have developed a special breed of transgenic mice that develops tau tangles from a human mutation, and can now test whether a specific compound might prevent tau tangles from forming in mice. Finding those successful compounds is crucial to developing therapeutics to treat diseases in humans, such as Alzheimer's disease, that have an important tau component to their pathology.

Dr. Lee is enthusiastic about the progress being made in their lab. "We have identified small molecules that inhibit the change in shape of tau in the laboratory," she told us. "That means we're on our way to testing a whole library of small molecules to see if they can inhibit tau tangle formation in an animal model. If we can do that, we will have something that could be used to treat people."

Looking for Other Roles of Tau

Dr. Lennart Mucke is the director of the Gladstone Institute of Neurological Disease and a professor of neurology and neuroscience at the University of California San Francisco. For many years, his primary research focus was the role of beta-amyloid in Alzheimer's disease and the role of another misfolded protein in Parkinson's disease. Findings from these studies have more recently led Dr. Mucke to take a close look at tau's role in AD. What he has discovered suggests that beta-amyloid needs tau to injure brain cells and that normal tau may play a role in regulating brain cell activity. In all these studies, Dr. Mucke and his research team have used transgenic mouse models and tissue cultures to study pathologic pathways and how this damage affects cells, networks of cells, and behaviors.

This tau story began in 2006, when Dr. Mucke's lab was doing a series of detailed studies of networks of neurons in transgenic mice that were bred to develop AD plaques. The team was surprised to find that beta-amyloid was stimulating nerve cells to send too many signals. Until this time, beta-amyloid had been known primarily for suppressing neuronal activity.

The lab found that when too much beta-amyloid was present, many more nerve cells than normal were mimicking the activity of other nerve cells. In other words, high levels of beta-amyloid induced abnormal neural network activity (or overexcitation) resembling epileptic seizures in learning and memory centers of the brains of mice. This type of epileptic activity could only be seen by brain wave recordings (EEG), but is similar to the EEG activity seen during twitching or other movements that occur in frank epileptic fits. "We began to suspect that some people with Alzheimer's disease may have similar hard-to-detect 'subclinical' forms of epileptic activity in

Dr. Lennart Mucke

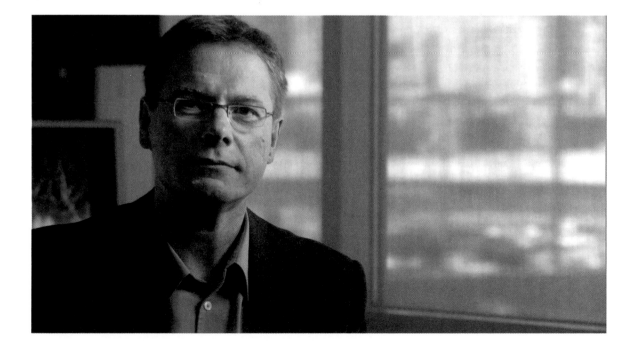

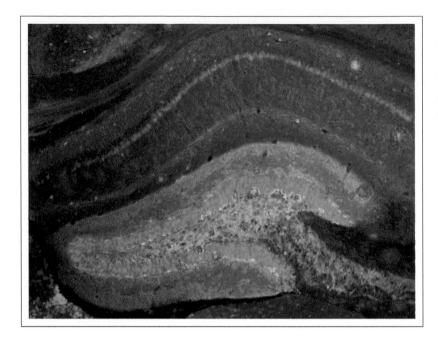

This brain section from a mouse bred to express the traits of human AD is stained to show amyloid plaques in red and neurons in green.

the brain and that this activity might contribute to their memory problems," Dr. Mucke said.

The overexcitation of nerve cells in the mouse models was followed by too little activity in the neural network, meaning that the brain went through waves of too much and too little activity instead of cruising along at a normal level. The period of lowered activity, which possibly occurred to cool down the hyperactive neurons, may also interfere with normal brain processes.

These findings may have been unexpected, but Dr. Mucke was ready to seize on the possibilities they presented to push the science forward. Because the elevated expression of tau increases risk for AD, he thought that network excitability might have some connections to the tau protein. "We wanted to know whether amyloid proteins could still overstimulate the nerve cells if we removed or reduced the tau protein." By selectively breeding transgenic mice, his team manipulated the levels of beta-amyloid and tau independently. Mice that had a lot of human beta-amyloid proteins in the brain and normal levels of tau had memory problems and neuron network imbalance. In contrast, mice that had a lot of human amyloid proteins but reduced levels of tau had normal memory and no network imbalance. "It was really striking to see mice whose brains were full of amyloid solve

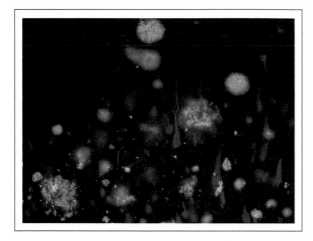

This microscopic slide of a brain section from a person with AD displays the classical hallmarks of the disease: beta-amyloid plaques (green) and tau tangles (red).

memory tasks without difficulty. Even reducing tau by only fifty percent effectively protected their cognitive functions against amyloid toxicity." Reducing tau also eliminated the abnormal network activity found in the amyloid-bearing mice. These findings contribute to some scientists' belief that the amyloid hypothesis is not a complete explanation for the dementia of AD.

The team then tested whether tau reduction had benefits even if there was no buildup of amyloid proteins. Using drugs that induce epileptic seizures to overstimulate the nerve cells of mice with no amyloid proteins, they found that reducing tau levels made the mice much more resistant to seizures. "Tau seems to regulate how much the nerve cells can be excited. If you reduce tau levels in a nerve cell, the amyloid proteins and other toxins can no longer push it into overdrive."

"Our findings are really encouraging. They suggest a strategy for protecting the brain from amyloid proteins and, perhaps, other disease-causing agents." Dr. Mucke's task now is to examine if tau reduction is safe when implemented in adult mice and to translate his discoveries into the development of drugs that can modify the levels of tau in humans or simulate the beneficial effects of this intervention.

3

DIAGNOSING EARLY MEMORY LOSS

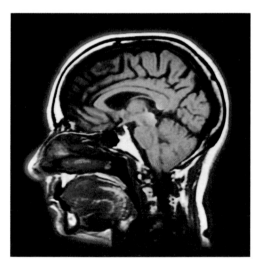

For years Alzheimer's disease could not be diagnosed until the person died and an autopsy
revealed an abundance of plaques and tangles
in the brain. However, scientists and clini-
cians around the world have been developing effective techniques to diagnose
AD even in its early stages. The diagnostic approaches consider a range of factors, including the results of physical exams, changes in performance on peri-
odic neuropsychological tests (tests that measure memory, language and math
skills, and other cognitive abilities), subtle changes in behavior over time, and

sometimes brain scans. (Part II of this book will explore recent advances in this area.)

Today, neurologists can be fairly confident of a diagnosis of clinically probable Alzheimer's disease. Studies have shown that specialized memory centers or doctors experienced in neurodegenerative diseases can diagnose AD with up to 90 percent accuracy, an impressive feat considering the complexity of the disease and the fact that, in the early stages, it can be difficult to distinguish from other types of age-related cognitive decline.

Diagnostic techniques are so important because the earlier that physicians diagnose AD, the better they may be able to treat the symptoms and track the disease process. Early diagnosis can also help spur people with memory problems to make the most of their abilities and interests while they still can. It also helps their families adjust to changing roles and realities and plan for the future.

Neurologist **Dr. Ron Petersen** has been a pioneer in classifying and diagnosing different forms of early-stage memory loss. He is the director of the Mayo Clinic's Alzheimer's Disease Research Center in Rochester, Minnesota, and Jacksonville, Florida. The Mayo Clinic center is one of a network of twenty-nine Alzheimer's Disease Research Centers around the country funded by the National Institute on Aging and specializing in research on Alzheimer's disease.

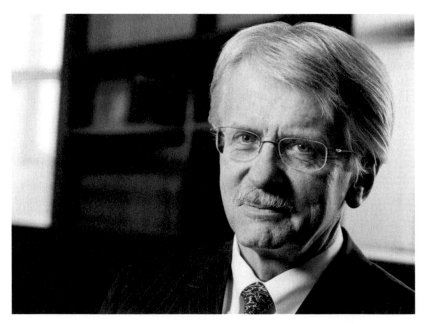

Dr. Ron Petersen

Back in 1994, Dr. Ron Petersen and colleagues at the Mayo Clinic diagnosed the beginnings of Alzheimer's disease in former president Ronald Reagan. President and Mrs. Reagan were open with each other—and the public—about the fact that the former president's forgetfulness was an early stage of AD. "This diagnosis was important to them. They felt that for the community and for the world at large, their recognition might show that if the president of the United States can develop Alzheimer's disease, anybody can. By encouraging people not to ignore possible signs of change, they made an important contribution to society," says Dr. Petersen.

Mild Cognitive Impairment

Because the onset of AD is so slow and symptoms develop gradually over many years, there is a period during which people are slightly more forgetful than they used to be, and perhaps more forgetful than they ought to be. They don't yet have other cognitive or behavioral problems that would classify them as having AD, however. This is the condition that Dr. Petersen named mild cognitive impairment, or MCI. Classifying this condition has been a major boon to researchers because it has provided the parameters within which to study subtle changes in memory and other cognitive skills that may predict the development of AD.

Long-term studies at the Mayo Clinic's Alzheimer's Disease Research Center and with thousands of other research volunteers around the world suggest that people diagnosed with MCI will go on to develop dementia (usually Alzheimer's disease) at a rate of 10–15 percent a year. "We need to identify these people at this earlier stage so that therapies and interventions can be designed to prevent that progression," Dr. Petersen told us. "Ultimately we'd like to identify people who are at risk of developing Alzheimer's disease and other diseases when they still have no symptoms."

Since first describing the condition, Dr. Petersen and other researchers have developed a framework for understanding the causes and consequences of MCI by identifying subtypes. These subtypes are based on the most affected cognitive skills, which may reveal the areas of the brain that are affected as well. Amnestic MCI, the subtype in which memory problems are the most important feature, indicates possible involvement of the hippocampal formation, the memory center of the brain. Other types of MCI, called nonamnestic MCI, are characterized by declines in other cognitive skills, suggesting damage to other brain regions. For example, some people may have difficulty processing visual information or trouble orienting themselves in space. They may be unable to reproduce a drawing or an arrangement of colored blocks. Such deficiencies suggest that other neurodegenerative diseases, such as frontotemporal dementia, as well as vascular conditions, might be causing this nonamnestic MCI.

The classification of two types of MCI—amnestic and nonamnestic—has been widely adopted by AD researchers and investigators conducting AD clinical trials. This framework may have a broader application as well. An understanding of amnestic MCI, combined with other diagnostic tools currently in development and drugs now undergoing clinical trial, may eventually help physicians diagnose and treat people before full-blown Alzheimer's disease has developed.

How Much Forgetting Is Too Much?

Dr. Petersen says, "It's not always easy to differentiate forgetting a friend's name from pathological forgetting. One of the most difficult questions we get is, 'How much forgetfulness is too much?'"

Consider the forgetfulness that many people experience as they age. A man comes home, flips his keys on the counter, and then can't find them five minutes later. A woman misplaces her reading glasses or her checkbook. She can't come up with the name of a coworker in the elevator. Three floors later, of course, it comes to her.

This kind of incidental forgetfulness isn't too serious. Age-related memory changes are very common and most often not related to a disease process. As we get older, we have to pay more attention or focus more on certain activities. It gets more difficult, for example, to drive and talk on a cell phone at the same time, because neither activity is getting our full attention.

On the other hand, if a person finds that he still cannot remember an experience even when he is focusing on it, that may be a sign of concern. If he forgets things he used to remember fairly easily, it may be a red flag. "You have a doctor's appointment next Tuesday because you think you're having side effects with your blood pressure medicine," Dr. Petersen suggested. "Tuesday comes and goes. You don't show up. That can happen every now and then, but when it happens today and it happened three weeks ago and you're afraid it's going to happen two weeks from now—and your family is starting to notice—that's when you may need to speak to somebody about whether the forgetfulness is more than age-related memory loss."

The key question is whether behavior has become different from usual. For example, someone who has always calculated the tip on a restaurant check asks another person to do it. Someone uncharacteristically wants to get his tax returns done by an accountant after taking pride in doing them for years, or asks someone else to drive because he can't remember how to get to a very familiar destination.

Based on the results of a physical exam and tests of memory and cognitive skills, the doctor may decide that the memory problems are not a concern. On the other hand, the doctor may decide that the changes are a sign of amnestic MCI.

Diagnosing MCI

In order for memory problems to point in the direction of Alzheimer's disease, the symptoms must be progressive. Therefore, in order to

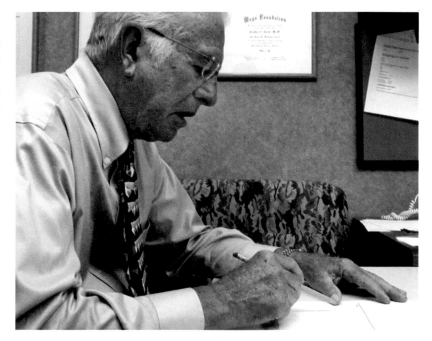

An important component of the current method of diagnosing AD is cognitive testing, which consists of memory and thinking tasks that can help distinguish dementia from the memory problems of normal aging.

diagnose a person, the doctor needs to establish a baseline level of ability, and then have the person come back some months later to see if performance declines.

Dr. Petersen's diagnostic approach to MCI includes a range of tests and activities to measure a person's cognitive abilities over time. He described how this works by telling the story of a man named Mr. Braun. When Mr. Braun first went to see Dr. Petersen, the team at the Mayo Clinic went over his entire medical and medication history. They also spoke to his wife to get her perspective. They performed a clinical examination in the office, which included physical and neurological tests and a mental status test. Based on those tests and on Mr. Braun's family history of Alzheimer's disease, they referred him for more detailed neuropsychological testing. These tests of memory and other thinking skills gave them a good profile of his cognitive performance.

"We saw that he did poorly on the paragraph recall test (a test in which a person listens as a paragraph is read to them and then is immediately asked to recall as many details as possible about it). In addition, when the team showed him a list of words to remember, he learned them fairly well, but thirty minutes later he could recall only one or two. We have information on how a person of Mr. Braun's age and general educational background should perform on these instruments, so we could compare him to normal people of his age. That led us to conclude that he was functioning at a lower level than we would expect for his age and background. We looked for other possible causes of the impairment—medical problems, medications, things of that nature that might have created this problem. There was nothing else, so we concluded that this was most likely MCI caused by a degenerative condition."

Sometimes doctors at specialized clinics perform other kinds of diagnostic tests, such as an MRI (magnetic resonance imaging), which reveals the structure of the brain, or lab tests to assess hemoglobin, vitamin B-12, and thyroid functions. These tests are useful because they can point to or rule out other conditions that may be contributing to memory problems. In some research centers, though not yet in medical practice, there may be a spinal tap to collect cerebrospinal fluid or other types of imaging scans of the brain.

Over the last three or four years, Mr. Braun's condition has gradually deteriorated. Mrs. Braun said, "He had been in contact with many individuals over his life, and he always remembered their

A Different Diagnosis

A diagnosis of MCI or Alzheimer's disease includes ruling out other possible causes of dementia. There are diseases other than AD that impair thinking and affect daily function, but the symptoms vary and may have a different cause. Different abnormal proteins are deposited in different parts of the brain, creating distinct symptoms. In AD, the abnormal proteins in plaques and tangles form in the memory parts of the brain first, and a person becomes forgetful. In the disease called dementia with Lewy bodies, different protein deposits are found in areas that control sleep, attention, concentration, and visual-spatial skills. Frontotemporal dementia involves the frontal and temporal lobes, which help control our ability to regulate our own behavior. A person with this form of dementia might exhibit behavioral abnormalities, inappropriate behaviors, and personality changes.

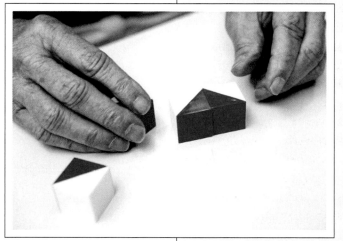

Dr. Petersen described the diagnosis of a person with nonamnestic MCI. The man came into Dr. Petersen's clinic with a range of problems. Although forgetfulness was an issue, it wasn't at the heart of his concerns. He was having difficulty focusing. He noticed that his mind would wander in conversation. He would turn to his wife and say, "What did he say?" He also noticed that when he would tell a story or talk to someone he would find himself thinking, "I'm not sure what my point was." When Dr. Petersen's team evaluated him in the laboratory, they found that the man had problems with attention, speed of processing, concentration, and visual-spatial ability. He was also having what is called dream enactment behavior. He would wake up in the middle of the night, flailing his arms and screaming, because in his dreams he was being chased by a dog or a car. In fact, one night his movements became so violent he fell out of bed and cut his scalp.

He was diagnosed with dementia with Lewy bodies, not AD.

Exercises where a person must copy a pattern, such as with these colored blocks, are also used during cognitive testing to help distinguish AD from other causes of dementia, some of which may affect visual perception.

names. But now, he's starting to forget recent acquaintances, people with whom he has had enough contact that he should have remembered them easily."

Each time Dr. Petersen has seen Mr. Braun, the symptoms have been a little more pronounced. His most recent exam told Dr. Petersen that Mr. Braun is progressing from MCI to AD. "An isolated occurrence is not a problem. But when it occurs on a repeated basis, when he is now forgetting events, items, information, names of people that he formerly remembered quite easily, this becomes a cause of concern." Dr. Petersen evaluated him further, and found not only a gradual decline in memory function, but also impairment in other areas of cognition.

"His executive function, his ability to pay attention, maybe his reading and writing skills, have declined such that it's not an isolated memory impairment any more. This is now a more widespread cognitive impairment." As the team talked to Mr. and Mrs. Braun about his daily activities, they could see that this was affecting his life. "He can no longer organize activities. He told us that he was helping his son build their home. A few years ago, he would have been the supervisor. Now he calls himself the worker bee. His son tells him, 'Cut here. Cut there. Get this. Get that,' because Mr. Braun can no longer put together the bigger, conceptual picture."

Dr. Petersen and his staff have worked hard to help the Brauns anticipate when Mr. Braun would cross the threshold to AD. "We've tried to prepare him for the fact that there's an increased probability of developing Alzheimer's disease when you have a family history and MCI," Dr. Petersen explained. By maintaining his intellectual and physical activity and staying involved with the family, Mr. Braun can help himself remain quite functional for as long as possible.

The Importance of Early Detection

Dr. Petersen explained to us why identifying cognitive decline at the MCI stage is so important. "We're trying to draw the distinction between those individuals who will not decline at all throughout life—so called successful aging, those who might experience a little bit of forgetfulness but not really progress to MCI or Alzheimer's disease, and those who ultimately will develop the disease."

A population study at the Mayo Clinic suggests how many

people may currently be at the MCI stage but don't know it. Dr. Petersen's team conducted a study of aging looking at a random sample of two thousand people in Olmsted County, Minnesota. Study participants ranged in age from seventy to ninety. Study investigators assessed how much cognitive impairment existed in this population. They found that more than 72 percent are aging normally. Though they may have a little forgetfulness, by and large they're functioning well. However, a little less than 17 percent meet criteria for MCI. About another 11 percent have some form of dementia, mostly AD.

"If we extrapolate this to the general population, up to thirty percent of all the people who are aging are at risk of developing cognitive impairment and Alzheimer's disease. These are astronomical numbers of individuals. We have a mandatory responsibility to diagnose these conditions as early as possible, and more importantly, to develop effective therapies that prevent cognitive erosion down the road," he said.

The current treatment options for Alzheimer's disease may help people function better for a few weeks or months or years, but they do not cure the disease, stop the underlying disease process, or prolong life in any significant way. Once memories are lost to AD, they can never be regained. That's why the key to effective treatment will be in early detection. "The earlier we intervene with therapies, the greater likelihood we will have of preventing the disease from developing. Prevention is where we need to go with this disease. It's too late if we wait until people have symptoms. So we really need those definitive biomarkers and clinical predictors of who's going to develop the disease in the future. Maybe it's going be a blood test. Maybe a cerebrospinal fluid test. Maybe an imaging test will tell us that a person has the propensity for developing Alzheimer's disease ten or twenty years in the future."

The Alzheimer's disease research community has already launched many clinical trials and other studies that they hope will make significant inroads against this disease. "We're on the threshold of making significant treatment discoveries," Dr. Petersen told us. "We're light years ahead of where we were in 1994 when former president Reagan came to the Mayo Clinic. In the last five to ten years, we've made enormous strides in understanding the biology of Alzheimer's disease. We know which abnormalities in the brain are likely causing the symptoms of forgetfulness and difficulties with daily activities. We know where they are in the brain and how they got there.

We have animal models for the disease and therapeutic models that can actually stop the disease process in animals. We have targets. The trick is to develop interventions that are going to stop the abnormal proteins from being deposited in the brain or clear these proteins from the brain.

"I hope that in my career I will be able to sit with a patient and say, I think you have the earliest stages of what might become Alzheimer's disease in the future, and here's what we can do about it."

DETECTING SUBTLE CHANGES

Neurologist **Dr. John C. Morris** is the principal investigator of the Alzheimer's Disease Research Center at Washington University in St. Louis. His team performs a wide range of clinical, cognitive, and other testing to diagnose the illness. The group's approach of conducting semi-structured interviews with patients and someone who knows them well (typically a close relative) has been credited with detecting dementia at its earliest symptomatic stages. The information obtained through the interviews is organized with the Clinical Dementia Rating (CDR). This scale, which was originally developed by Dr. Leonard Berg, Dr. Charles Hughes, and others at Washington University and later refined by Dr. Morris, is a five-point scale that determines the presence or absence of dementia and, when present, its severity. A zero on the scale indicates no cognitive impairment and the other four points connote very mild, mild, moderate, or severe dementia. The CDR has been widely adopted nationwide and abroad as a global measure of dementia.

Dr. Morris's diagnostic approach is based on whether a person has declined in cognitive or other abilities in relation to that person's previously attained levels. To determine whether individual decline has occurred, Dr. Morris's team not only examines the person

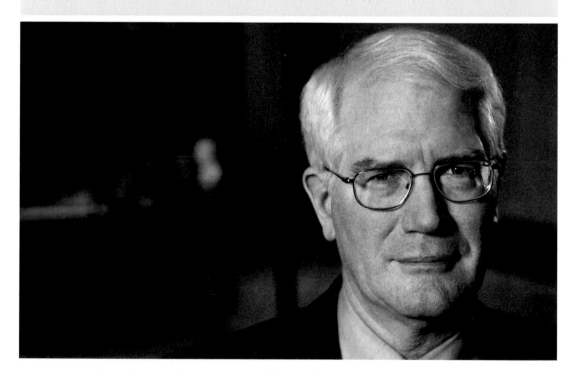

but also carefully interviews someone else. "Typically, this is the spouse, an adult child, or other family member, but it could also be a colleague or a neighbor." Most important to Dr. Morris's team are the insights that family members or close friends can provide on how a person is performing now in relation to his or her previous abilities. A person in the early stages of AD may appear healthy to a casual observer, may be unaware of mild deficits, and may still perform reasonably well on formal tests of memory and thinking, so the observations of someone who can describe how he is doing now in comparison with his prior performance are needed to detect the illness.

"From a memory and thinking standpoint, older adults who are aging normally remain independent. They still make their own decisions, remember everyday tasks such as taking their medications, and perform accustomed activities, all without unusual reliance on others. It may take them longer to recall details and they may use memory aids such as lists to help, but basically they remain independent. When a person begins to decline, and the family is called on more and more and more to help out, that's a clear warning sign."

Dr. Morris agrees with the recommendation to seek help when early changes in behavior or memory begin, even if they seem quite mild. For example, a person who has always prepared her own income tax return might be struggling with it now. If there are sufficient subtle changes that seem to be consistent and progressive and come to the attention of family and friends, a medical evaluation is in order. Because they have an intimate knowledge of a person and her behavior, family and friends can play an important role in identifying potentially problematic changes in memory or cognitive ability, and they are in a unique position to act on that knowledge to get help for the person. "Even though we do not yet have a cure or prevention for Alzheimer's disease, it's important to seek evaluation and management right from the beginning to determine whether it possibly is Alzheimer's disease or if there is another explanation. If Alzheimer's disease is suspected, symptomatic therapies are available that can benefit the patient, at least somewhat. Most importantly, at the early stage the patient can be involved in decision making about her future."

Many matters can be arranged in advance of the disease's more debilitating phase. Does the individual have a durable power of attorney? Who will she assign that to? Should she continue to live in her home or should she choose an alternative? What about driving? Is there a need to supervise medications? Who will manage her financial matters? This is the time when she and her family can decide these things, rather than waiting until a guardian must be appointed to speak for her.

One woman came in to Dr. Morris's clinic with her adult son. When Dr. Morris interviewed the son alone, he heard much concern. One problem was she was constantly unplugging electrical devices and her phone lines. "I don't know what's going to happen tomorrow morning if I leave her at home tonight. I can't even call her." The son was obviously alarmed at the changes in his mother's behavior. Dr. Morris used this information to determine how much she had changed from before, and that helped him understand whether these changes were abnormal.

In a separate interview, Dr. Morris asked the mother her age. She said, "Isn't it terrible when somebody forgets her own age? I was born in 1930."

He persisted. "So roughly, if you had to guess, how old would you say you were?"

She answers, "I'm seventy-four." Actually, she is seventy-eight.

After many other tests, Dr. Morris concluded that she likely has mild dementia caused by Alzheimer's disease. He gave her and her son the results of the tests and his diagnosis, emphasizing that it is relatively early-stage and there is much that she can still contribute to herself and her family. He suggested that she remain physically, mentally, and socially engaged, and reviewed safety and security issues at home. Dr. Morris suggested that she and her son avail themselves of the information and support provided by the Alzheimer's Association. Finally, he recommended that she begin one of the approved drugs to treat the symptoms of mild-moderate Alzheimer's disease, although he noted that the drug is not a cure and ultimately will not change the disease outcome.

Dr. Morris enjoys answering questions from patients and families and is gratified by how frequently the family rises to the considerable challenges of caring for people with dementia. "It is remarkable how often family members, individually and collectively, accept the burdens necessary to provide truly loving, supportive care. I am inspired by their devoted caregiving, but I hope one day that we can develop truly effective therapies that not only treat the symptoms of Alzheimer's disease but also can be used as prevention to stop this illness from ever happening."

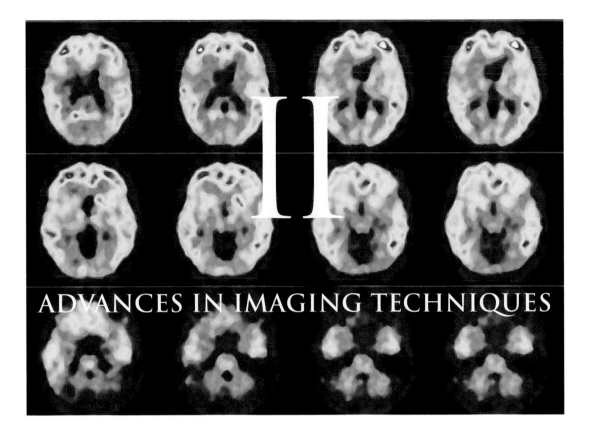

II
ADVANCES IN IMAGING TECHNIQUES

S ome have called this time a golden age of neuroscience. Advances in many areas, from molecular biology to genetics, have accelerated the pace of discovery far beyond what could be imagined a few decades ago. Behind many of the advances have been new technologies for imaging the brain.

When Dr. Alzheimer first described this devastating brain disease, he relied on findings from a microscopic examination of a patient's brain tissue after she died. From that time until the 1980s, the brain with Alzheimer's disease remained a black box. Scientists could only see the characteristic brain pathology at autopsy. The development of magnetic resonance imaging (MRI) and positron emission tomography (PET) has transformed neuroscience. Scientists can now see the size and structure of discrete parts of the living brain and can visualize brain function during cognitive tasks like reading or solving math problems. Even more importantly, they can track changes in brain structure and function over time, and compare images with the results of traditional paper-and-pencil tests of memory and cognition. A world of knowledge has opened up, bringing new possibilities for diagnosis, identifying targets for drug therapies, and suggesting methods for monitoring response to interventions.

Types of Neuroimaging Scans

Several different neuroimaging techniques have become the mainstays in AD research.

Magnetic resonance imaging (MRI) uses magnetic fields to generate clear computer images of internal structures in the body. MRIs can image the brain and provide a detailed picture of the brain's anatomy. Scientists use them to measure the size of brain structures. MRI tests have been used extensively in AD research to track which regions of the brain are atrophying and filling with fluid as AD progresses and to understand changes in brain structures like those in the hippocampal formation.

A functional MRI (fMRI) is used to measure brain activity during a mental task, such as one involving memory, language, or attention. Researchers can measure the functioning of the brain regions engaged in those tasks. Several scientists, including one we'll meet in the next chapter, are using fMRI to visualize functional changes that suggest the brain tries to compensate for the damage that occurs during the AD process.

A positron emission tomography (PET) scan uses a small amount of short-lived radioactive material coupled to another molecule to look for functional change in the body. The material travels through the blood and is concentrated in organs and tissues. The PET machine then measures the energy given off by the radioactive tracer and converts it into three-dimensional pictures that can be viewed on a computer screen. PET scans of the brain are used heavily in AD research because they can show how well discrete areas of the brain are

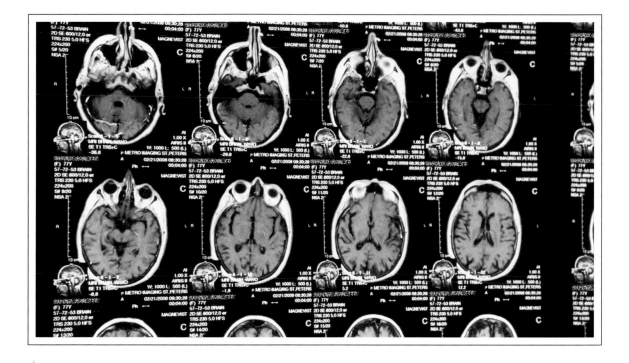

This series of cross-sectional brain images was produced by MRI.

functioning. PET is now being used with a radioactive tracer called Pittsburgh Compound B (PiB), which attaches itself to beta-amyloid in the brain. The vibrantly colored PiB images, which are generated by computer analysis, reveal concentrations of beta-amyloid in areas of the brain. This allows researchers to correlate beta-amyloid deposition in living individuals with memory loss or other cognitive or biological changes.

Alzheimer's Disease Neuroimaging Initiative

Recognizing the promise of neuroimaging for Alzheimer's disease research, the National Institute on Aging launched the Alzheimer's Disease Neuroimaging Initiative (ADNI) in 2004. This five-year, $60-million public and private partnership is the largest AD initiative ever and is primarily funded by the National Institutes of Health.

Dr. Richard Hodes, the director of the NIA, explained the groundbreaking nature of this initiative. "NIA scientists involved in AD research and pharmaceutical and biotechnology companies all realized that we very much needed to develop a systematic approach to studying normal older people, people with Alzheimer's disease, and people with MCI through the use of neuroimaging techniques and testing of biochemical markers such as molecules found in blood or cerebrospinal fluid. But we had to conduct this research in a way that could be carried out in multiple centers across the country, that could use standards agreed upon by all, and that ultimately could be used by the research as well as the pharmaceutical community. This great need led to the development and funding of the Alzheimer's Disease Neuroimaging Initiative."

This initiative, a financial and intellectual partnership of private-sector entities coordinated through the Foundation for NIH, involves the National Institutes of Health, the Alzheimer's Association, the Food and Drug Administration, and scientists in the U.S. and Canada. The initiative has been following two hundred cognitively healthy older individuals and four hundred people with MCI for three years, and two hundred people with early-onset AD for two years. By taking MRI and PET scans at regular intervals, ADNI researchers hope to learn when and where brain changes specifically related to Alzheimer's disease occur and how the disease progresses.

The imaging information is being correlated with the results of both neuropsychological tests and analysis of blood, urine, and cerebrospinal fluid. Both the imaging and fluid biomarkers can provide indications of the progression of disease over time.

Traditionally, research centers collect and analyze data from imaging and biomarker testing in a variety of ways, and on smaller groups of people. By standardizing the process across the fifty-seven participating research sites and pooling all the findings, the initiative hopes to provide data that will indicate which biomarkers, or combinations of biomarkers, can most reliably predict the progression of cognitive decline, MCI, and AD. These markers could then be incorporated into clinical trials funded by the federal government and the pharmaceutical industry. Such standardization would reduce the cost and length of drug development trials.

During the first several years, ADNI researchers set up the study's research structure, enrolled participants, and began collecting data. These data are now coming in for analysis. An important characteristic of the initiative is that the clinical, neuropsychological, imaging, and biological data collected are available to all qualified scientific investigators as a public research resource. This has fostered cooperation and cross-pollination of ideas in the field and is serving as a model for research on other diseases and for other AD researchers. In fact, similar AD neuroimaging research efforts have been launched in Australia, Japan, and Europe.

The high-powered scientific expertise that is being brought to the Alzheimer's Disease Neuroimaging Initiative is a major reason for the excitement that this initiative is generating. Another aspect, less discussed but equally compelling, is the commitment of the people who are volunteering their time and energies as participants. It is no surprise that people with AD and MCI are committing themselves to this effort. However, study participants with normal cognition are just as important to the research efforts. Dr. Charles DeCarli, a neurologist at the University of California, Davis School of Medicine and an ADNI team leader, described their significance this way: "ADNI's success depends on the people who are participating. They're coming from all over the United States and Canada. They are really committed, not only for three years, but to have pencil-and-paper testing and MRIs and PET scans multiple times, blood samples, and repeated lumbar punctures. So why are these people doing it? I think some of them do it because they know someone who has Alzheimer's disease, and they understand that we're trying our best to use this information to design new treatments. Some of them are doing it because they recognize that Alzheimer's disease is a major problem in our society and is only get going to get worse. They are contributing their time and energy to benefit science."

.   .   .

Part II moves beyond the basic science of Alzheimer's disease to look inside the diseased brain. As Dr. Scott Small of Columbia University Medical Center put it, "The history of medicine really can be tracked according to technical innovations that have allowed us to visualize disease in a living patient." The next chapters explore how some recent technical innovations in neuroimaging are contributing to this golden age of AD research. These technological milestones may be particularly valuable for studying the earliest brain changes that lead to AD. Once scientists understand how the disease process begins and are able to track its progression in individuals, diagnosis will become more accurate and drug development more fruitful.

Chapter 4 tells the story of the critical discovery of PiB, the radioactive tracer used with PET scans to show the distribution of beta-amyloid plaques in a living person's brain. More than a century after this disease was first identified, researchers are only now able to watch it run its destructive course inside an individual's brain, instead of having to wait until autopsy to see the damage. Chapter 5 features two scientists who are using MRI and fMRI to pinpoint the regions of the brain where AD begins and study how the cognitive decline of AD differs from the memory loss associated with normal aging.

4

VISUALIZING PLAQUES IN THE LIVING BRAIN

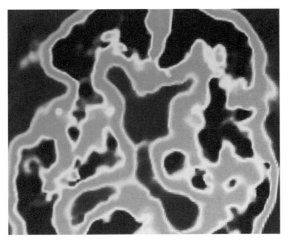

It may seem far-fetched to imagine looking deep into the brain tissue of a living person and seeing whether beta-amyloid plaques are there. If you could do that with a person who has the clinical features of Alzheimer's disease, you would not have to wait until an autopsy to diagnose the disease definitively. This would have a huge impact on early and accurate diagnosis, on tracking the progression of the disease, and on monitoring responses to drugs and other treatment interventions.

Currently, clinicians must rely on cognitive tests both to diagnose Alzheimer's disease and to follow its progression in people who have it. These exams are not only time-consuming, but they also require a highly trained person to conduct them and a practiced clinician to interpret the results. Beyond the practical concerns, an individual's results on a cognitive test can vary greatly over time—even though the overall cognitive decline associated with Alzheimer's disease progresses steadily over the years, a person's function can vary on a daily basis, and neuropsychological exams are unable to take those short-term swings in performance into account. Even more important, the very nature of cognitive tests ensures that they will not detect the disease until clinical symptoms are present.

Over the past fifteen years, many scientists sought to develop a more accurate, consistent, and strongly correlated biological measure of a person's cognitive decline to help make a more definitive diagnosis. This chapter tells the story of two scientists whose hard work and discoveries led to the development of the tracer compound that may make this possible. The very first scan images using their compound in a living human brain showed the same distribution of beta-amyloid that is typically seen on autopsy in cases of Alzheimer's disease—plaques high in some areas and low or even nonexistent in others. For the research team that had worked for years to develop this imaging technique, seeing these images was a jaw-dropping moment. They knew instantly that this technique would forever change the way Alzheimer's disease would be studied.

The radioactive tracer compound they discovered, Pittsburgh Compound B, or PiB, is injected intravenously prior to a PET scan of the brain. PiB binds to beta-amyloid plaques in the brain, and not to parts of the brain that are free of plaques. A PET scan using PiB will produce an image showing where in the brain the beta-amyloid deposits are concentrated.

Dr. Richard Hodes, director of the National Institute on Aging, gave us some context for the significance of PiB's discovery. "We are looking to designs of newer, more specific, and more sensitive criteria for diagnosis and monitoring. In the field of neuroimaging, perhaps the most prominent example of late has been Pittsburgh Compound B. We have, until this time, been looking at the effect of Alzheimer's disease by looking at loss of brain volume and brain cells, or looking at gross changes in the metabolism of cells in the brain. The ability to monitor lesions that may be more directly involved in the pro-

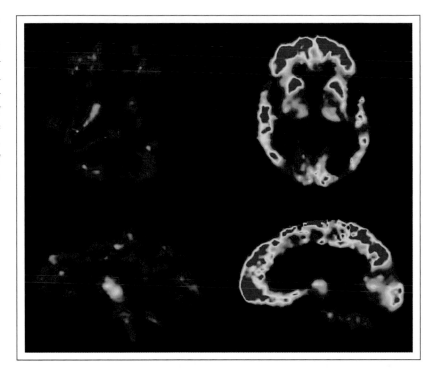

PET scans showing PiB retention—and thereby beta-amyloid deposition—in the brains of a cognitively healthy person (left) and a person with AD (right). The greater the presence of beta-amyloid, the more red and yellow appear on the PET scan.

gression of the disease process would be an enormous advance. And Pittsburgh Compound B, which is capable of directly identifying, monitoring, and tracking changes in the beta-amyloid protein, one of the hallmark lesions of Alzheimer's disease, represents such an example."

A Shared Dream

The story of the discovery of PiB starts with the frustration of many scientific groups around the world. For more than a century, the only way to diagnose Alzheimer's disease definitively was to examine a person's brain tissue after death to see whether the brain showed the characteristic hallmarks of the disease—plaques, tangles, and extensive brain atrophy. In a living person, the best that could be said was that the person had "probable Alzheimer's disease," meaning that they had the typical history, signs, and symptoms of Alzheimer's disease, and that no other explanation was likely.

Scientists knew that excess beta-amyloid was a key feature and requirement for the diagnosis of the disease, but they were able to identify brain beta-amyloid deposits only in the brains of people who had already died. The identification of beta-amyloid was done with the use of chemical agents that bound to beta-amyloid in a tissue section of the brain stuck to a glass slide. If they could use similar chemical agents to see beta-amyloid in the brain of a living person, it would be a major step forward, not only in terms of improving the accuracy of diagnosis but potentially for developing new drugs. The difficulty was developing an agent that would work in a living person—binding specifically and selectively to beta-amyloid in such a way that scientists could measure the amount in the person's brain and also make sure it left the brain safely, after a short time.

Enter **Dr. William Klunk,** a neuropharmacologist and professor of geriatric psychiatry, and **Dr. Chester Mathis,** a chemist and professor of radiology. Dr. Klunk and Dr. Mathis were strangers working in different specialties and in different parts of the University of Pittsburgh School of Medicine before they began their collaboration. They were introduced by a senior faculty member who felt they had similar research interests, and they discovered a shared goal: utilizing the imaging potential of radioactive compounds seen in PET scans to visualize amyloid plaques in the living brain.

Dr. Klunk's research had been focusing on compounds that bind

Dr. William Klunk and Dr. Chester Mathis

▼

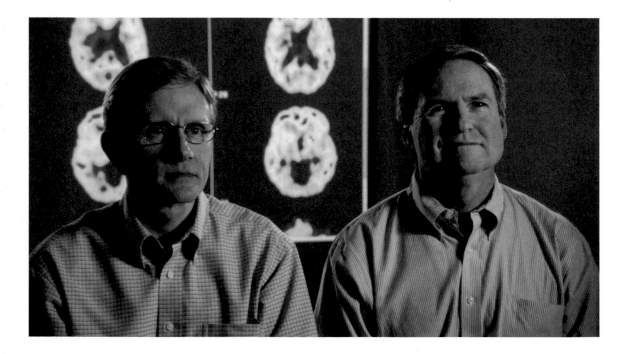

to beta-amyloid. Since the late 1980s, Dr. Klunk had been working with a compound called Congo red, a dye that pathologists use at autopsy to stain beta-amyloid plaques for viewing under the microscope. When he arrived at the university's PET facility to meet with Dr. Mathis, he discovered that Dr. Mathis had also worked with this compound. In the mid-eighties, Dr. Mathis and several neurologists at the University of California Berkeley had tried unsuccessfully to get this dye past the blood-brain barrier, a protective barrier in the brain's blood vessels that prevents charged or large molecules from entering the brain. Dr. Klunk suggested working with other, more brain-penetrating, versions of Congo red that might enter the brain more readily than Congo red itself and show beta-amyloid plaques using a PET scan. Dr. Mathis was very interested.

Glue and Glitter

Developing this compound was fraught with difficulties. It took eight years and many dead ends. Dr. Klunk and Dr. Mathis's first challenge was to make a compound that could penetrate the blood-brain barrier and bind to beta-amyloid in high concentrations so that it could be seen after the rest of the compound had been cleared from the brain. The team worked on a group of Congo red derivatives for about six years. They made hundreds of variations, but they were just short of their goals. In these disappointments they saw opportunity. The many unsuccessful attempts helped them understand exactly what properties they were looking for. Feeling that they had exhausted this group of compounds, they decided on a new approach and began to look at a group of dyes that were totally different in structure from Congo red.

They chose to try radioactive versions of thioflavin dyes, another class of chemicals that bind to beta-amyloid that have been used for many decades to study brain tissue of people who have died of Alzheimer's disease. The first animal studies showed that radioactive thioflavin dye derivatives crossed the blood-brain barrier easily, bound well to beta-amyloid, and did not bind to anything in the brains of normal control animals and thus were cleared rapidly from normal brain tissue. The researchers knew they were on the right track.

Within a year, Dr. Klunk and Dr. Mathis were ready to test the compound in humans. In 2001, there was no fast-track mechanism to evaluate new PET imaging compounds in the United States, but one was available in Sweden that could save the researchers valuable research and development time. Years earlier, colleagues at Uppsala University in Sweden had agreed to help the Pittsburgh team in their research by being objective testers for their compound. In mid-2001, Dr. Klunk and Dr. Mathis chose a compound to send to their Swedish colleagues. This first compound was dubbed "Pittsburgh Compound A" by the Swedish team. But before PiA was ever tried in humans, Dr. Klunk and Dr. Mathis made one more change and sent a second compound to their Swedish colleagues, thinking it would be superior to PiA, although it was only subtly different. The Swedes dubbed this second compound "Pittsburgh Compound B"—or PiB.

The doctors received a call from Sweden on Valentine's Day 2002. They were told, "This is a sweet day. We have reason to celebrate." The Swedish group had done the first PET scan with PiB on a person with Alzheimer's disease. Later they did the same with other people with Alzheimer's disease and with cognitively healthy people. The results were just what they were hoping for. Dr. Mathis told us, "The healthy people didn't retain much PiB, but the patients with Alzheimer's disease had a lot."

Dr. Klunk explained how PiB works by comparing it to a craft his children enjoyed while growing up. "My kids would take a piece of white paper and draw something on it with white glue. (Think of the glue as beta-amyloid.) Then they would sprinkle glitter all over the paper. (Think of the glitter as PiB tracer.) It's a big, glittery mess. You don't know what's glue and what isn't." Then the kids would turn the paper upside down and shake it. "Everything that wasn't stuck to the glue fell off. When the kids turned their paper right side up, they could see the design they made out of glue and glitter on a background of white paper."

Just as the glitter shakes off the part of the paper not covered with glue, blood in the brain washes the PiB tracer that's not stuck to the beta-amyloid out of the brain. "When we do PET scans with PiB, we get pictures that are specific to exactly what we're looking for."

Dr. Klunk and Dr. Mathis cleared a huge hurdle when they developed PiB, but another obstacle faced them. Images from the first PiB scans revealed patterns of beta-amyloid deposition that were very similar to those typically seen in people who had died of Alzheimer's disease, but the team couldn't be absolutely sure that the PiB binding was accurate until they could compare PiB scans from a group of individuals against the results of autopsies after those same individuals had died.

Six years after the first PiB scans, enough time had passed that the researchers were able to examine the donated brains of several people who had had PiB scans during life. Working with Dr. Klunk and Dr. Mathis, a team of researchers in Pittsburgh led by Dr. Milos Ikonomovic and **Dr. Steven DeKosky,** a leader in the field of Alzheimer's disease and former director of the University of Pittsburgh's Alzheimer's Disease Research Center, saw a very close correlation between beta-amyloid plaques seen on the PET scan using PiB and amyloid plaques detected upon autopsy. This was evidence that the PET scans were, in fact, imaging beta-amyloid in a living human brain, and that the levels they had measured in life were representative of what they had measured at autopsy.

In 2008, the American Academy of Neurology awarded Dr. Klunk and Dr. Mathis the Potamkin Prize for their discovery of PiB and the outstanding contribution to the study of Alzheimer's disease and related dementias that it represents.

Research volunteer with early-onset AD undergoing a PET scan with PiB to track the progression of beta-amyloid plaque accumulation in his brain.

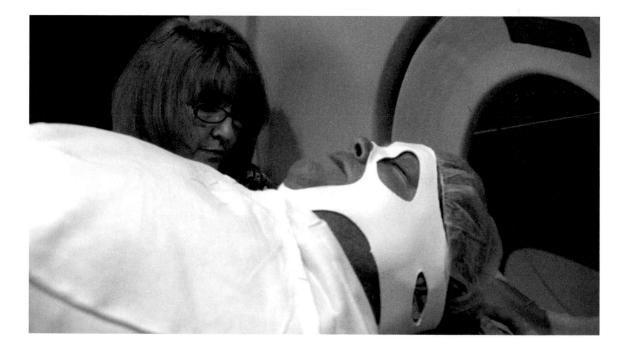

Applications Present and Future

Not surprisingly, as the initial PiB images began to be shown publicly to the scientific community, they generated tremendous excitement. "Everyone wanted to get their hands on PiB," Dr. Mathis told us.

Once a connection between PiB levels and cognitive decline has been correlated and clinically defined, it may one day be possible that PET scans with PiB will become a tool that experienced physicians and memory clinics use to diagnose Alzheimer's disease or to identify people who are likely to develop the disease in the future. But there are challenges to address before that can happen, with issues for patients and in technical aspects of performing the scans routinely. First, optimal use in a clinical context would depend on proof that the amyloid hypothesis is correct and that a disease-modifying treatment that lowered brain beta-amyloid levels would result in cognitive stabilization or improvement.

Further, even if doctors were ready to use PiB clinically, a simple technological issue would still pose a big problem. PiB labeled with carbon-11 is a short-lived radioactive compound that must be used immediately after it is created in a cyclotron. Ninety percent of PET scanners around the country that could use the PiB tracer cur-

Scientists manufacture PiB in a sealed room using robotic arms to prevent unnecessary exposure to radiation.

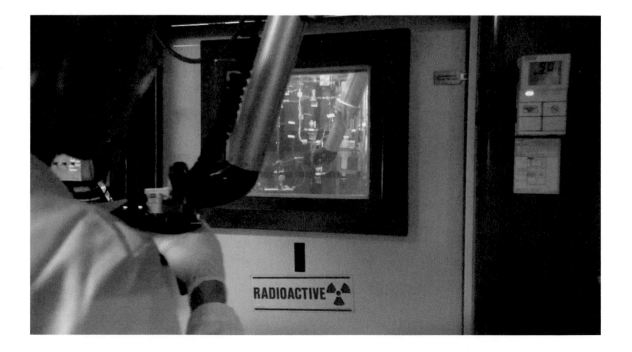

rently don't use it because the hospitals and research institutions where the scanners are located cannot produce it. A longer-lived radioactive compound that could be shipped to distant hospitals and researchers is needed so that PiB could be used more widely in PET scans. Work is proceeding now on radio-labeling PiB with other tracers such as fluorine-18 that will maintain their active state for a longer time. Once this is achieved, the tool may become more widely available. Dr. Mathis estimates that such a variant of PiB is three to five years away, depending on FDA approval.

The Alzheimer's Disease Research Center at the University of Pittsburgh School of Medicine is facilitating the use of the current PiB compound by the broader scientific community. When the university licensed the commercial development of PiB to a private corporation, it stipulated that the short half-life version (the type that wouldn't be developed for commercial use) would be provided free to any university around the world who wanted to conduct research with it. PiB is currently being used for Alzheimer's disease research in more than forty institutions around the country and the world.

In the years since PiB was discovered, it has quickly become apparent that this imaging technology can make many valuable contributions to our basic knowledge of Alzheimer's disease and our efforts to address its devastating effects. PiB is helping scientists answer a long-standing basic question about beta-amyloid plaques and normal cognition. Even before the PiB studies, it was well known from autopsy studies that people could be cognitively healthy but still have an abundance of beta-amyloid plaques in their brains. Scientists had different explanations for this seeming paradox. "There were two camps," Dr. Klunk explained. "One said, 'There are amyloid plaques in the brain of a cognitively normal person. This means the plaques occur very early and precede all the other changes that lead to Alzheimer's disease and memory loss.' But the other camp said, 'Here's a cognitively normal person with a brain full of beta-amyloid plaques. That means plaques don't always cause cognitive impairments.' The first camp replied, 'If they had lived long enough, we would have seen those cognitive impairments appear.'" The second camp argued that some brains, for as-yet-undetermined reasons, have the ability to withstand the presence of plaques, a concept known as "brain reserve."

This argument has not yet been settled, but Dr. Klunk believes that PiB is a tool that will help settle it. "We have identified cognitively normal people—about one in four seventy-year-olds—who have beta-amyloid plaques in their brains. We can now see these plaques in people during life, and we're actively following them over time. Colleagues at other institutions are actively following others as well. We'll be able to see if they can live ten years without ever having cognitive problems and developing memory loss. Will some fraction of this 25 percent of seventy-year-olds become the eighty-year-olds who have Alzheimer's disease? We finally have the tool to answer that question." In essence, PiB could serve as a marker for the development of Alzheimer's disease in the brain over time. Findings from these and other PiB studies will help researchers understand more fully the complex trajectory that takes a person through all the stages from a healthy brain to a brain with Alzheimer's disease. Investigators will also be able to compare these inside-the-brain PiB findings with outward, clinical signs of memory loss and cognitive change that can be tracked through observation and paper-and-pencil cognitive tests. This will give them an even richer understanding of the disease process and suggest ways that an individual's overall health, lifestyle, and life experiences may influence that process.

Continuing on work begun with Dr. DeKosky and the University of Pittsburgh Alzheimer's Disease Research Center, Dr. Klunk and Dr. Mathis are also applying their PiB scan research in studies of MCI. The Pittsburgh team is finding that, in scans of individuals diagnosed with MCI, many of the subjects—but not all of them—have plaque deposits. Since not all people with MCI develop Alzheimer's disease, the scan may help predict which people with MCI will develop Alzheimer's disease and which have another cause of memory loss. This could prove very helpful in deciding which people with MCI to treat with drugs designed specifically for Alzheimer's disease.

The use of PiB scans may also help to accelerate the rate of drug development. Dr. DeKosky explained this potentially important contribution of PiB. Many of the drugs that are now being developed and studied in animals and people target beta-amyloid in one way or another. Current prescription therapies can alleviate symptoms for months to years, but they do not seem to alter the underlying disease process. The goal of all ongoing drug development and the proof of a drug's effectiveness will be whether it can slow down or stop the loss of memory and cognitive function in humans. In the past, when researchers tested medications on people, they had to follow their research volunteers for many years to determine whether the progression of Alzheimer's disease symptoms had slowed.

By using PiB with PET scans at regular intervals throughout the drug testing, researchers would be able to see what effect the drug was having in the brain within a shorter timeframe. "If we give someone a medication that we expect should either stop the progressive accumulation of beta-amyloid plaques or decrease or remove them, we can see much more quickly whether beta-amyloid is removed by scanning someone with PiB six months or a year after they've started their medications," Dr. DeKosky explained. If the scan shows good results, and the person is performing significantly better than the people in the trial who didn't get the active compound, "We'll know the drug is a winner. Someday, scientists could identify people in their fifties or sixties who have positive scans but who are otherwise healthy. They could give medications that would forestall Alzheimer's disease so that these people wouldn't develop the disease until they were a hundred years old. That would be a very fine target."

Dr. Dale Schenk, a researcher at Elan Pharmaceuticals on the front lines of AD drug development, described the potential impact that PiB may have on clinical trials over the coming years. "What it means is that for any treatment we can ask, 'In patients who are treated with it, does the amount of plaque they have in their brain go down?' We don't have any results yet. But we think that's going to be

Dr. Steven DeKosky

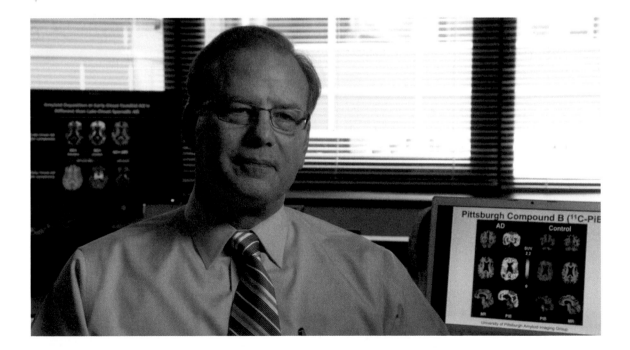

very important. I anticipate that, if a future experimental treatment is working, we very well might see a reduction in PiB labeling, or plaque labeling, when we image the brain during the clinical trial. This is a fantastic tool, because all of us researchers in the field can now ask many more questions about what's going on with plaques. Do they get worse as the patient progresses? Do they get better? We'd love to know about that."

5

APPLYING NEW TECHNOLOGIES IN RESEARCH

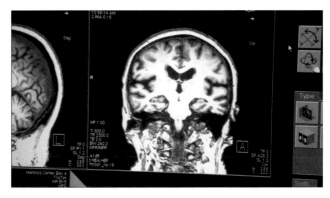

For many Alzheimer's disease researchers, the ultimate goal is to identify the first step that transforms a healthy aging process into the inevitable cascade toward Alzheimer's disease—in other words, to understand when the pathology of AD begins to affect actual brain function. Can we discover the earliest changes in memory and cognitive function that signal to us that all is not well? To answer that question, we need to know how to measure brain function and how to recognize the early signals of dysfunction.

Dr. Reisa Sperling, of Harvard University, believes she may have found methods to detect early signals of brain trouble. Dr. Sperling studies how people form and retrieve memories and why this fails in the earliest stages of AD. Her studies, which take advantage of recent advances in MRI and PET scan technologies, suggest that certain areas of the brain involved in creating and retrieving new memories may go into a kind of overdrive in early AD. She hypothesizes that this change in function may be a harbinger of cognitive decline.

Dr. Sperling first became interested in AD when her grandfather developed serious memory problems the year before she started medical school. "Here was a man who'd always been the intellectual leader of our family, who'd always been able to teach me and my father. To see him requiring help with dressing and feeding was heartbreaking. The first time I visited him that year, he still remembered who I was and was able to interact with me. But by the end of the year, he knew I was someone he'd seen before, but he didn't remember my name or who I was. It was so painful to see the disease rob him of his identity. As much as I try to stay objective with my patients, when I encounter that loss and remember what it was like for my grandfather. . . . I don't think you ever get over it."

Today, Dr. Sperling hopes that her findings and those of others

Dr. Reisa Sperling

▼

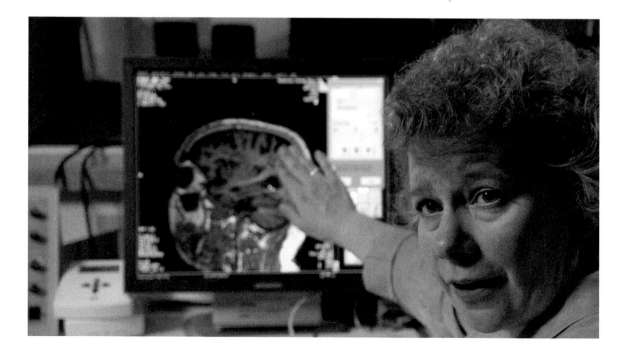

will help researchers and clinicians identify people at high risk of developing AD before the disease has set in fully, so that interventions can begin early, when they may have a better chance of minimizing or, one day, even stopping the disease process.

Watching the Brain Create Memories

The brain stores information in a cohesive way so that we can recall the myriad of details about an event: who was there, what music was playing, what the food smelled and tasted like, how the occasion made us feel. These aspects of an event are bound into an integrated "memory trace" so that the whole event can be retrieved instantly. In order to store and retrieve information, the brain has to perform three functions. First, information that has been learned only moments earlier is captured in short-term memory. Next, the brain moves the information into long-term storage. Finally, the brain has to be able to find and retrieve the memory on demand.

One of the brain regions involved in moving information from short-term memory to long-term storage is the hippocampal formation. Scientists have studied individuals who have had extensive damage to their hippocampal formation; the moment their attention is diverted, they have no memory of a conversation they've been having. A person with a malfunctioning hippocampal formation would still have lots of thoughts and would be able to perform activities, but wouldn't be able to form new memories or learn new facts.

Using functional MRI (fMRI) scans, Dr. Sperling has focused on a network of brain regions that are involved when a person is engaged in forming a memory. The scans clearly show that these regions engage in a finely tuned process in which one area turns on very rapidly when a person is learning something new. That region, the hippocampal formation, is responsible for binding new information together into a short-term memory, which can later be transferred into a long-term memory for storage in other brain areas. At the same time, other areas of the brain, in particular the parietal regions, must turn off so as not to interfere with the memory formation process. Later, when the person recalls a memory, the process is somewhat reversed. Many of the regions in the brain that were turned off during memory formation now turn on to retrieve the memory. This cycle of turning on and turning off, or activation and deactivation, as Dr. Sperling called it, happens all the time.

"When we look at the fMRI of a healthy person, we see that the memory network is carefully synchronized. The parietal regions are constantly turning on and off and working in coordination with the hippocampal formation. This network activity correlates with how well the person is able to perform the memory task."

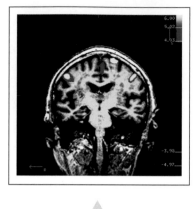

In a person with Alzheimer's disease, the fMRI shows little or no activation of the hippocampal formation when the person is asked to learn something new. This correlates with pathological changes in the brain, as this area is among the first to be damaged in AD. Dr. Sperling explains that MRI scans of people with Alzheimer's disease show shrinkage, or atrophy, of the hippocampal formation as well as a thinning of the brain or loss of neurons in the parietal regions. The parietal regions are also especially vulnerable to the formation of beta-amyloid plaques in AD.

The colored areas of this fMRI scan show brain activity in a person with AD.

Dr. Sperling is now conducting fMRI studies that use face-name memory to see whether beta-amyloid is causing these disruptions in the activation and deactivation process in people with early-stage AD, as well as to study those with MCI and normal memory function. While conducting an fMRI study, Dr. Sperling asks research volunteers to look at photographs of faces and learn to associate each face with a name. The face-name recognition task is particularly difficult for people with AD, which is why she chose it for the test. "If you want to determine whether someone is at risk for a heart attack, you put them on a treadmill and stress the system. We stress the brain with memory tests to see how it performs."

While lying in an fMRI machine, research volunteers are shown many pairs of face photos labeled with names. Thirty minutes later, they are shown the same faces with two name choices and asked to recall the name that goes with each face. This fMRI technique allows Dr. Sperling to see which parts of the brain are activated and deactivated during the exercise. A healthy person would quickly form the association between the photograph of a face with the name Bill, and the fMRI would indicate that normal hippocampal activation had occurred during that formation of a face-name association for Bill. On the other hand, when a person with AD tries to learn the Bill face-name association, the fMRI scan shows little or no activity in the hippocampal formation and they might look at Bill's picture and say, "It could be Bill or Jim. I have no idea."

One of many cards used in the face-name test.

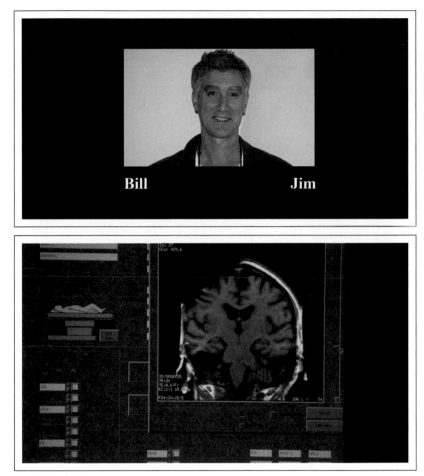

An MRI image taken during the face recognition study.

A Hyperactive Hippocampal Formation

Dr. Sperling was surprised to see that some people in the study with mild memory problems had an extremely active hippocampal formation when they were trying to process a new memory. This suggested to her that, in these people, the hippocampal formation might have been trying to compensate for the damage done by the advancing Alzheimer's disease process. In people with mild cognitive impairment, thought to be a precursor stage of AD, the hippocampal formation may be going into overdrive. "It works harder to form a new memory. It's revving and driving as fast as it can." During that phase of hyperactivity, people are able to maintain memory. Unfortunately, hyperactivity doesn't continue, and Dr. Sperling hypothesizes that it may be a sign of impending failure of the hippocampal formation. "More and more, we've seen that hyperactivation is a strong predictor of who is going to decline over the next two years. Before the hippocampal formation fails, it seems to make a last-ditch effort to activate as much as it can, struggling to form memories."

The brain works hard to compensate for the damage resulting from many neurodegenerative diseases, such as Huntington's disease, Parkinson's disease, and stroke. In people with AD, the ability to compensate may last for only a short time. Dr. Sperling has observed in her recent studies that memory tends to decline rapidly in the year or two after the hyperactivation phase.

Dr. Sperling has followed fifty people over time, including healthy people and those with MCI. The same face-name task was conducted during an fMRI session at two-year intervals. The healthy people showed no difference in the activity of their hippocampal formation. In some of those with MCI, this activity didn't decline much over the two years. But those individuals whose initial scans displayed hyperactivation of the hippocampal formation showed deterioration. "About half of the people in this third group had developed clinical Alzheimer's disease over these two years."

Dr. Sperling's team is now scanning older people every six months with fMRI to track brain function and using PET scans with PiB imaging to detect beta-amyloid plaque formation, as well as to see if there is a correlation between plaque formation and fMRI hyperactivation. Such a connection might have important implications for both diagnosis and drug development. If Dr. Sperling and other researchers are able to establish a definitive link between hippocampal hyperactivation and the impending onset of clinical Alzheimer's disease, fMRI scans of the hippocampal formation could be used as a predictive biomarker to aid physicians in diagnosing the disease and in selecting subjects for clinical trials who are well matched for the potential outcome of the trial. Ultimately, this type of information could be used to start treatment at an earlier stage of AD—a refinement that is much needed.

An Even Closer Look

Dr. Scott Small is taking a very close look at one of the key phenomena of Alzheimer's disease: how the disease spreads from its first site of damage in the hippocampal formation to engulf the entire brain.

Dr. Small told us, "One of the basic tenets in clinical neuroscience is that diseases, no matter how complex, start in one part of the brain and then spread over time. To get an accurate snapshot of the early stages of a neurodegenerative disease like AD, you must follow people at the very beginning. But you don't really know who has the disease then."

One reason it's hard to know who has the disease is that the early stages of AD are characterized by a subtle problem that Dr. Small calls "cell sickness." A scientist looking at the brain tissue of a person who died after many years of AD will see clear evidence of extensive cell death—the brain tissue has atrophied and the fluid-filled spaces in the brain are greatly enlarged. In contrast, nerve cells are still present during the earliest stages of AD. They are not functioning very well, but they haven't yet died. "It turns out to be quite challenging to actually visualize the cell sickness stage using conventional imaging techniques."

As a result, investigators are conducting long-term studies that follow hundreds of healthy elders, using a variety of imaging and other tests to capture the cell sick-

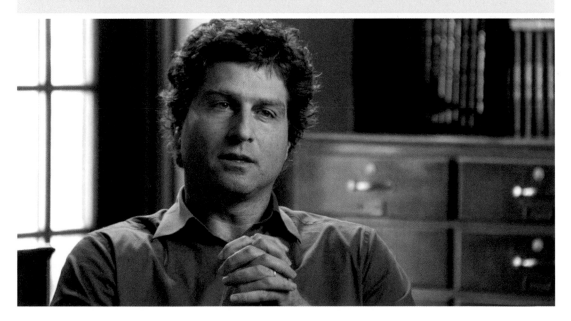

ness stage of the disease and determine when the disease really begins. "If we could capture that stage of the disease it would offer a lot of hope for better treatment. After all, it's easier to treat a sick cell than a dead cell."

In his search to capture the cell sickness stage, Dr. Small is focusing on the function of a small part of the hippocampal formation called the entorhinal cortex. His work to pinpoint the first signs of disease poses a real challenge, however. "One of the earliest symptoms of Alzheimer's disease is mild forgetfulness, which implicates the hippocampal formation. We can document that with neuropsychological tests. So the question is why can't we take any sixty- to seventy-year-old with memory changes and just call that early AD? The reason we can't do that is because normal aging itself will also affect memory and hippocampal function."

Dr. Small and his research team are trying to resolve that diagnostic dilemma by focusing on the microanatomy of the hippocampus. They want to know whether the earliest stages of AD and normal aging may affect memory function differently because they act on different areas of the hippocampal formation. This possibility makes sense because these structures are "not just a collection of homogenous, look-alike neurons. Different regions contain neurons that have different physiological and molecular properties."

He began these studies by modifying imaging techniques so that he could study this microanatomy. He had several requirements. The technique had to be sensitive enough to detect cell sickness before cell death occurred. The imaging technique also had to have very high spatial resolution, because the areas are just a few millimeters in size. Finally, the technique had to work with animals as well as humans, so that the hypothesis could be tested more easily. Dr. Small wanted to start the research with mice, which have a hippocampal formation similar to our own.

After six years, Dr. Small and his team had an MRI scanner that met their needs. He can now visualize minute sections of both the human and the mouse hippocampal formation, each containing a unique population of cells. His research team has been working with AD transgenic mice and humans to test the hypothesis that Alzheimer's disease and memory changes in normal aging affect different brain subregions.

Dr. Small's modified MRI creates maps of the brain. On the computer screen, he color codes regions to show levels of function. Cooler colors like blue indicate relatively low activity, while warmer colors like red show more, or relatively normal, function. On his scans, the entorhinal cortex of people—and mice—with AD show up as blue areas of dysfunction. In people who are aging normally, the same areas appear red.

Dr. Small pointed to an fMRI image and explained. "Evidence appears to be emerging that the entorhinal cortex shown here circled in red in both the human and

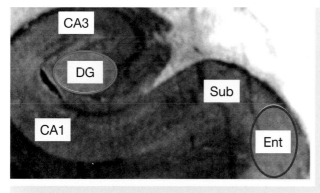

mouse hippocampal formation seems to be affected first and foremost in AD, but not exclusively. Ultimately, other areas are also involved, but this is the area that's most vulnerable to the disease. In contrast, normal aging seems to affect the area circled in green, called the dentate gyrus. Other studies have suggested this as well, but this is really the first time that we can begin to detect this pattern in living subjects. The ability to visualize this dysfunction, and to be able to do it across species, will help us achieve the goal of distinguishing the very earliest stages of AD from memory changes that happen normally in aging."

If Dr. Small's imaging findings are confirmed and expanded in additional studies by others, these techniques may eventually become a diagnostic tool that can help distinguish memory loss associated with AD from the forgetfulness that can come with healthy aging. The National Institute on Aging is currently providing his lab with funding to conduct these studies. He is imaging hundreds of healthy elders and following them over time. Some may develop AD, and many will not. "Can we detect the earliest stages of Alzheimer's disease based on these imaging studies? Only time will tell."

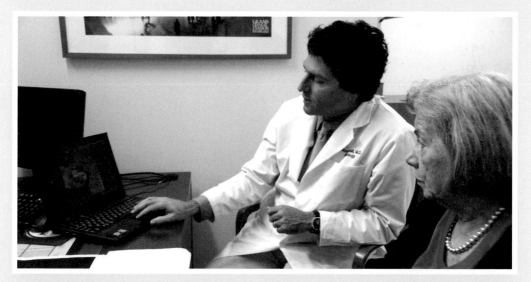

Dr. Small and a research volunteer review an fMRI image showing the functioning of her hippocampal formation.

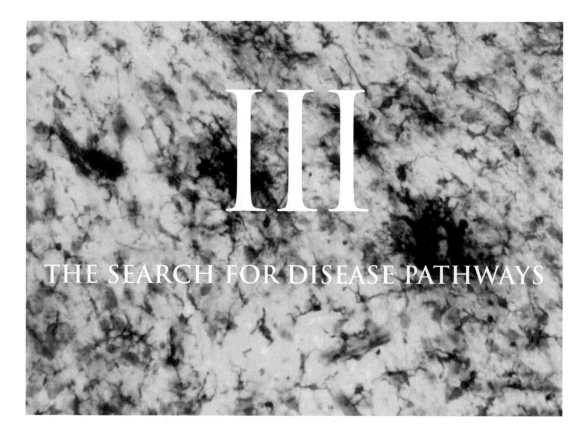

III

THE SEARCH FOR DISEASE PATHWAYS

What causes Alzheimer's disease? What starts and promotes the disease process that leads to an overabundance of beta-amyloid, a buildup of plaques and tangles, and loss of function and death among brain cells?

Scientists increasingly agree that there is probably no one cause of this most complicated disease. They are identifying and studying many contributing factors, including genetics, environmental and lifestyle factors, and connections with other diseases of the body.

Dr. Richard Hodes of the National Institute on Aging told us, "Since our understanding of the basic processes underlying the disease is still incomplete, science has to remain very open to multiple hypotheses. These are not competing hypotheses, because they may not be mutually exclusive."

One of the originators of the amyloid hypothesis, Dr. Dennis Selkoe, recognizes that many elements besides beta-amyloid are at work. "Alzheimer's disease is a multifactorial disease. Our current knowledge suggests that beta-amyloid is a necessary and sufficient factor for inducing the condition we call Alzheimer's disease. However, it has a lot of bad helpers. Targeting one of these helpers may have a powerful influence on risk—look at how much lowering LDL cholesterol in the bloodstream decreases the likelihood of heart attack or stroke."

Because the ultimate goal of medical research is the prevention and treatment of disease, it is important not to target just one cause or develop only one therapeutic strategy. Dr. Lennart Mucke said, "We should not put all our money down on one particular disease target, certainly not at this stage, when many clinical trials have failed. There is great reason for hope that recent insights will lead us to a combination of effective treatments. We need to support further research in many areas with more energy, more people, more programs, and more funding."

Part III looks at research that is illuminating pathways to AD and opening up possibilities for new therapeutic approaches.

Genetics

Genetics often plays a crucial role in helping scientists understand the underlying causes of a complex disease process, such as the one at work in Alzheimer's disease. If they can pinpoint the genetic mutations or variations that influence the development of a disease, either directly or indirectly, they can often work forward to find the proteins that the genes code for, and the metabolic processes that might be affected by them. In the AD field, breakthroughs in the knowledge of genetics have suggested many new avenues to explore with further research.

Chapter 6 features Dr. John Hardy, Dr. Alison Goate, and Dr. Gerard Schellenberg, who played prominent roles in the identification of two of the three genetic mutations that cause early-onset AD. We will follow the research that has led to the discovery of several such genes and explain how, even though early-onset AD affects only a very small number of families, the identification of those genes has had a tremendous impact on science's understanding of both early- and late-onset AD.

Vascular Disease

One of the most promising disease pathways scientists are currently investigating is an association with vascular disease. Epidemiological and animal studies have suggested that vascular disease may contribute to the development of Alzheimer's disease. This line of research is important because vascular diseases such as high blood pressure and heart disease are so common, and therefore may play a role in a great number of cases of AD. Scientists such as Dr. Charles De-Carli and Dr. Thomas Beach, both featured in Chapter 7, are excited about the opportunities that establishing a connection between vascular disease and AD may present, because it may be possible to reduce the risk of AD by treating vascular diseases concurrently. We know so much about the causes of vascular disease—as well as how to treat and prevent it—that definitively linking it to AD might lead immediately to the application of new therapeutic and preventative strategies.

Insulin Resistance and Diabetes

A third pathway to Alzheimer's disease may be diabetes and insulin resistance, the underlying condition that leads to diabetes. Epidemiological studies have shown that people with type 2 diabetes are at increased risk of cognitive problems, including MCI and AD, as they age. In Chapter 8, we look at this association through the work of Dr. Suzanne Craft. She has focused on insulin resistance, which precedes and characterizes type 2 diabetes, hypothesizing that insulin resistance damages the ability of the brain to form memories. Dr. Craft does not claim that insulin resistance is the only cause of AD. "Our thinking is that there are several important pathways to Alzheimer's disease, and this is one of them." However, her work is enormously important because nearly 20 percent of Americans over sixty have type 2 diabetes, and it is thought that even more have insulin resistance. These conditions, like vascular disease, can be prevented by exercise, diet, and other lifestyle changes.

Inflammation

Inflammation is one of the means by which the body's immune system reacts to the presence of toxic substances. Even though scientists may have originally considered it a bit unorthodox to approach Alzheimer's disease research through the lens of the inflammatory response, it is not altogether surprising that it seems to have an important relationship to the disease process. Chapter 9 looks at the work of Dr. Joe Rogers, who is studying the possible role of inflammation in AD, including a potential causal relationship between brain inflammation and beta-amyloid plaques. There is much we still don't know about inflammation in the brain, but since it is both a positive and negative process in the body, sorting out its role in AD will be a difficult task. This is yet another pathway that may lead somewhere unexpected.

. . .

Researchers are following all these pathways and more. Dr. Craft captured the importance and the challenge of keeping an open mind. "Simple answers don't translate well to this very complex disease. As the writer H. L. Mencken once said, if you give me a complicated problem, I can give you a solution that's quick and simple and elegant and wrong." She commented on how the multifaceted nature of Alzheimer's disease gives us a number of pathways to follow. "This is a time when we're going to learn a lot about what causes Alzheimer's disease, and aging itself."

6

DISCOVERING THE GENETICS
OF ALZHEIMER'S DISEASE

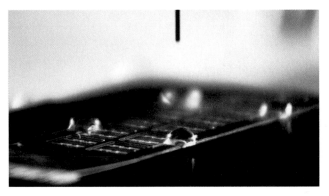

For more than a century, scientists have known that some people who die in middle age with memory problems and dementia have brains filled with beta-amyloid plaques and neurofibrillary tangles. Dr. Alzheimer had first identified this pathology in a woman in her early fifties, and, for decades, scientists thought that Alzheimer's disease occurred very rarely and only in younger people. Senility, on the other hand, was considered a normal part of aging.

In the 1950s and 1960s, pathologists began examining the brains of people who had died with senility in old age. To their surprise, they recognized that the brains looked like the one Dr. Alzheimer had described. They concluded that senility and Alzheimer's disease were the same condition. Their challenge became finding a common cause for two seemingly different disease processes with the same final pathology.

As research progressed in the 1960s and 1970s, scientists identified some families in which members of many generations had developed Alzheimer's disease at an early age—what we now call early-onset Alzheimer's disease. In these families, people who had a father or mother with AD appeared to have a fifty-fifty chance of getting the disease. This inheritance pattern is called autosomal dominant inheritance. Clearly, something in the genetic make-up made it likely that some family members would develop AD at a young age, usually between the ages of thirty and sixty.

In the 1980s, technological advances in genetics and computers made it possible to search for the genes that cause this form of the disease. Researchers collected and analyzed DNA samples from members of family groups in an effort to identify a mutated gene the affected relatives had in common and compare it to the same gene of unaffected family members.

Since then, patient, meticulous, and insightful research has begun to reveal the genetics of Alzheimer's disease. The search has involved some very special families, large research initiatives, advanced computers, and many brilliant scientists. So far, researchers have found three genetic mutations that lead directly to early-onset AD, as well as a genetic variation that has been confirmed to increase susceptibility to late-onset AD, which occurs in people aged sixty and older. This is the story of these important discoveries, which have many critical implications for treatment options as well as for our understanding of the disease process.

Genetics in Early-Onset AD

A breakthrough in the hunt for the first AD gene was made in London through the collaboration of **Dr. John Hardy** and **Dr. Alison Goate.** In 1985, Dr. Hardy received a letter from a woman in Nottingham, England. Her father had developed Alzheimer's disease in his early fifties. The family tree she included in her letter showed that four of her

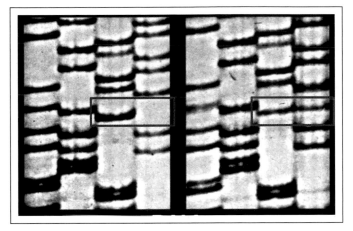

The image on the left shows the DNA of a normal individual, while the DNA on the right highlights the mutation in the APP gene that causes some cases of early-onset AD.

father's nine siblings also had AD. They were all alive and between fifty and sixty years old. She also had affected cousins; in a group of six siblings, three had AD.

According to Dr. Hardy, "Somewhere in this family's DNA, a mutation was causing this disease. We knew it had to be there because AD never skipped a generation." Dr. Hardy traveled to Nottingham to collect blood samples from the entire family. "We were on a quest to see which mutated genes had been inherited by this woman's father and the other affected family members, but not by others."

Other researchers had already discovered that a section of chromosome 21 contains the gene with the instructions for the formation of APP (amyloid precursor protein), which is embedded in the cell membrane and from which beta-amyloid is cleaved. "We went straight to that gene. Indeed, in this family, the APP gene containing the instructions for the APP protein was mutated in the affected individuals, but not in the other family members. The APP protein produced by the mutated gene had a perfect structure except for a single mistake,

Dr. Alison Goate

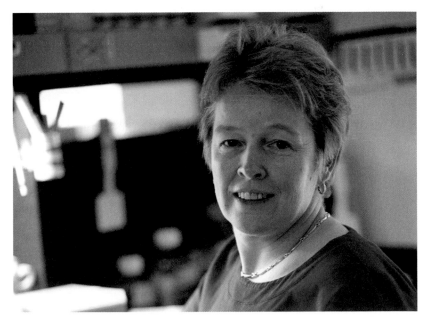

exactly where one of the enzymes that cleave the beta-amyloid out of the amyloid precursor protein does its work. We knew then what was going wrong in this family."

Finding this APP mutation took Dr. Hardy and Dr. Goate four years of painstaking work with genetic sequencing. When they discovered it, "It was a remarkable day," Dr. Hardy says. "This was going to change our lives. It was a fantastic thing to have worked out the genetic code in this family. The family was very proud of the finding, too. They went on national television to share how happy they were that they had contributed to the understanding of the disease."

It was a tremendous achievement—the first time a single, specific genetic cause for Alzheimer's disease had been found. But when researchers examined other families with a high incidence of early-onset AD, they did not find the same mutation in the APP gene. Apparently other mutations must also be possible, and some have since been found in other places in the genome. Eventually, through similar genetic sorting procedures involving other groups of volunteer early-onset families, a group of scientists led by Dr. Peter St. George-Hyslop, then at the University of Toronto and who now has a joint position at Cambridge University in England, identified another gene involved in inherited early-onset AD. This gene is called

Dr. John Hardy

▼

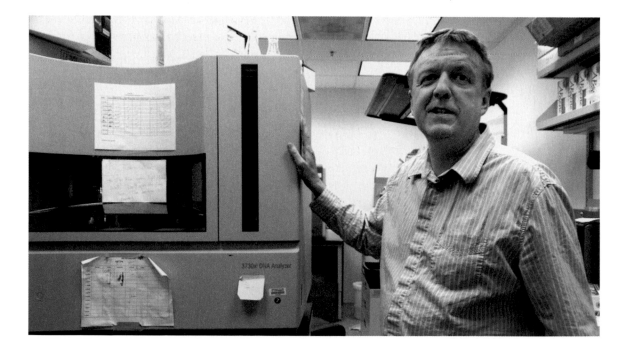

presenilin 1, and it resides on chromosome 14. Since its original discovery, large numbers of different mutations in the presenilin 1 gene have been identified. Some people with mutations in this gene develop an extremely severe form of AD in their late twenties.

Other groups with high occurrences of inherited early-onset AD were also found and studied. An extended family that proved especially valuable to the research was a group of Germans who had first settled in the Volga River region of Russia in the 1760s, then emigrated to the Midwest of the United States at the beginning of the twentieth century. Dr. Tom Bird, a neurologist at the University of Washington, heard about the high incidence of early-onset AD among a group of wheat farmers in that community. He began going from family to family asking, "What's your background?" After repeatedly hearing, "I'm from Russia but I'm not really Russian. I'm a German," Dr. Bird discovered that these different families with early-onset AD all had the same history. They had originally come from two towns only a few kilometers apart near the Volga River.

The frequency of early-onset AD among this population did not seem to be a coincidence. It seemed likely that the families were descendants of a single individual with a genetic mutation that caused early-onset AD. Dr. Bird's investigations of these ethnically German families from Russia led to the discovery of a third early-onset gene mutation—presenilin 2, which resides on chromosome 1. The discovery is credited to **Dr. Gerard Schellenberg,** who had been Dr. Bird's colleague at the University of Washington but is currently at the University of Pennsylvania; Dr. Rudy Tanzi at Harvard University; and their colleagues. Several different mutations in the presenilin 2 gene lead to the development of Alzheimer's disease in the mid-forties through mid-eighties. The people with early-onset AD in this group all have mutations in the presenilin 2 gene.

Significantly, all the mutations currently known to cause the inherited early-onset form of AD increase the production of toxic forms of beta-amyloid. These genetic findings showed that beta-amyloid is a critical player in the *development* of early-onset AD, not just an *effect* of the disease process.

Discovery of these genetic mutations also made it possible to make an animal model of Alzheimer's disease. As Dr. Goate describes the significance of these genetic discoveries, "For the first time, it actually was possible to think about making an animal model of Alzheimer's disease. Before that, there was no animal model, and it really impeded research." Today, animal models of AD—mostly mouse models with mutated human APP genes inserted into their chromosomes—are a mainstay of AD research and provide a valuable tool for exploring many biological questions.

Genetics in Late-Onset AD

The discoveries of the three genes responsible for early-onset AD were made at the same time that our understanding about the pathology of Alzheimer's disease was growing. By the 1980s, pathologists had concluded that the rare early-onset form of AD was, for all intents and purposes, the same as the much more common late-onset form—both exhibited the plaques and tangles, steady progress from cell sickness to cell death, and clinical features of memory loss and dementia. The linking of genetic mutations to beta-amyloid formation in early-onset AD suggested that genetics must be involved in the late-onset form as well, but that something other than dominantly inherited genetic mutations were at play. However, as Dr. Schellenberg describes, the science needed to identify the genetic factors that contribute to late-onset AD was much more complex to carry out than the search for the

Basics of Gene Sequences

DNA provides every cell with instructions for almost everything it builds and does. Located in the cell's nucleus, DNA is composed of four chemicals called bases—adenine (A), cytosine (C), guanine (G), and thymine (T). DNA is organized into intertwined strands called chromosomes, and each cell has 23 pairs of them. A chromosome contains thousands of segments called genes, each a specific sequence of bases. The sequence tells a cell how to make a specific protein. A permanent change in the sequence of bases in a gene is called a mutation. Even slight variations in the sequence may produce an abnormal protein that can lead to cell malfunction and disease. Other, more common variations in a gene's sequence of bases can increase the chances that a person will develop a disease without automatically causing it. When this happens, the gene is called a susceptibility gene.

Geneticists searching for the causes of a disease now have the tools to comb through and compare millions of gene sequences from people with and without the disease to find such variations. Scientists looking for genes associated with Alzheimer's disease often focus on the genes associated with proteins involved in Alzheimer's pathology, particularly APP, the amyloid precursor protein that is the source of beta-amyloid.

early-onset mutations. "Late-onset Alzheimer's disease did not give us a very clear picture of what inheritance had to do with the disease. So we focused on those early-onset families because we really knew how to handle those. We knew how to do the science to find the genes. Late-onset Alzheimer's disease has been much more difficult."

Fortunately, the work geneticists have done to understand early-onset AD has been of enormous importance to the search for the susceptibility genes that contribute to late-onset. "The vast majority of people who have Alzheimer's disease have late-onset Alzheimer's. But if we understand the early-onset, we understand these genes, we understand how they tie into the pathology, and we know that the pathology in early and late is very similar, then what we learn from the genetics of early-onset AD would also apply to the late-onset disease," Schellenberg said.

When scientists began to search for these weaker genetic links to late-onset AD, they found no clear inheritance pattern. They began to suspect that many genes might be having small effects on the series of events that cause the degeneration of healthy neurons due to beta-amyloid plaques and tau tangles. In this scenario, they conjectured, genetic variations would not cause late-onset AD, but would increase the likelihood of developing it.

Dr. Gerard Schellenberg

▼

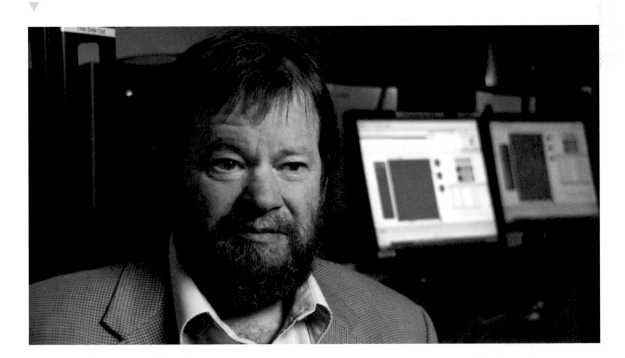

"We're looking for risk genes," Dr. Hardy explained, "genes that could influence amyloid metabolism. Our challenge is to understand what predisposes people to typical late-onset AD. We expect there to be a mixture of predispositions, some environmental and some genetic." A similar mix of risk factors plays a role in other disorders like Parkinson's disease and type 2 diabetes.

There is an intense hunt to identify these risk-factor or susceptibility genes. Scientists are deciphering DNA profiles of thousands of research volunteers, comparing patterns in the genes of people with AD to the genes of people who don't have it. When they find such patterns in the DNA of people with AD, researchers study that particular gene sequence. What chromosome is it on? What genes are in that area, and with what genes do they interact? What proteins do they code for? These proteins then become targets for further study.

One susceptibility gene on chromosome 19, called ApoE, was identified by Dr. Warren Strittmatter, Dr. Allen Roses, and their colleagues at Duke University. This gene contains the instructions for apolipoprotein E, a protein that carries cholesterol from cell to cell, and within cells, both in the brain and in the rest of the body. (Brain cells use cholesterol to repair membranes and carry out normal functions.) This connection to cholesterol has significant implications for understanding how Alzheimer's disease and vascular disease are related, a subject that will be explored at length in the next chapter. Intriguingly, it also holds potential for the treatment of AD, since cholesterol is such a well-understood molecule.

In humans, the three ApoE alleles or variants are: ApoE-ϵ2, ApoE-ϵ3, and ApoE-ϵ4. We're each born with a combination of two of these, one inherited from each of our parents, i.e. ApoE-ϵ2-ApoE-ϵ2, ApoE-ϵ2-ApoE-ϵ3, ApoE-ϵ2-ApoE-ϵ4, etc. Each combination has a different effect on susceptibility to AD. The relatively rare ApoE-ϵ2 appears to provide some protection against AD. The most common gene, ApoE-ϵ3, appears to have no effect on AD risk. But ApoE-ϵ4 increases a person's risk of developing AD, and people with two ApoE-ϵ4 alleles tend to develop AD at an earlier age. However, since this is not a gene that causes disease directly, unlike the early-onset mutations, some people with ApoE-ϵ4 may never develop AD. Conversely, the fact that some people who develop the disease have ApoE-ϵ2 or ApoE-ϵ3 tells researchers that other susceptibility genes besides ApoE-ϵ4 are likely to be at work.

At the same time, in Dr. Schellenberg's words, "better, newer, fancier technology" is helping geneticists track down still more susceptibility genes. "Today we can look not just on every chromosome or every section of every chromosome, but almost every unit of DNA. For less than four hundred dollars, we can test five hundred thousand to a million sites in one person's genes on a computer chip the size of a postage stamp." With this technology, AD researchers believe it's only a matter of time before they find more susceptibility genes.

One of the most influential research endeavors in recent history is the Human Genome Project. Since scientists succeeded in sequencing the human genome in 2003, identifying all the approximately 20,000-25,000 genes in human DNA, a vibrant new generation of genetics research is under way. Geneticists around the world are now able to employ the data from the Human Genome Project in a research method called genome-wide association studies (GWAS). These studies allow scientists to associate different gene variations with observable traits, such as the presence of a disease like AD. GWAS require thousands of participants belonging to two groups: people with the disease and people without the disease, similar in age and other related factors, to act as controls. Scientists obtain samples from each participant and then scan each participant's genome for genetic variation. If a certain genetic variation appears more frequently in

Dr. Schellenberg's team extracts DNA from blood samples for analysis. The DNA is visible as strands suspended in the golden liquid.

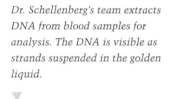

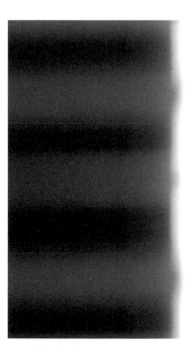

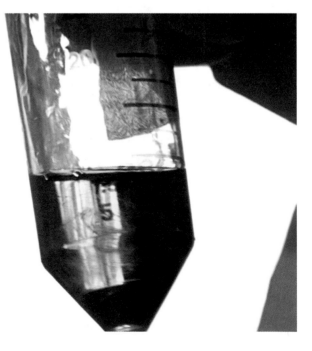

people with AD, that variation is said to be "associated" with the disease and provides researchers with a clue that a susceptibility gene that increases a person's risk of developing Alzheimer's disease may reside in that section of the genome. This allows researchers to focus on the most promising genes in an unbiased fashion.

What Is My Risk?

Dr. Schellenberg is often asked, "My father or mother has Alzheimer's, so what's my risk?" Unfortunately, at present, neither he nor other researchers have easy answers. Since late-onset Alzheimer's disease is not caused by a dominantly inherited mutation, it is impossible at this point in time to calculate someone's risk. However, people have so much concern about their chances of developing this disease that scientists apply the knowledge gained from population studies to derive rough estimates of risk. Such population studies have suggested two factors that contribute to an increased risk of developing AD: whether an individual has an affected first-degree relative, such as a

---

Huge Genetics Initiatives

Scientists need many DNA samples to find more susceptibility genes for late-onset Alzheimer's disease, identify possible environmental influences, and understand the interplay between the two. The advances in science enabled by the completion of the Human Genome Project in 2003 and the development of the GWAS technique inspired the NIA to launch an initiative to identify at least 1,000 families that have members with and without late-onset AD. Investigators in this Alzheimer's Disease Genetics Initiative are collecting blood samples and other clinical data from these volunteers. Researchers expect that DNA analysis of these samples will help us understand the genetics of Alzheimer's disease more thoroughly and find additional susceptibility genes.

In 2007, the NIA created another new program—the Alzheimer's Disease Genetics Consortium—to facilitate collaboration among leading researchers. Its goal is to gather much of the DNA that has already been collected by scientists around the country into a single study, supplement it with samples from some newly recruited participants, and then to scan those thousands of genomes for AD susceptibility genes and other genes connected to age-related cognitive decline. Many volunteers are needed to participate in this project and other studies like it. Dr. Schellenberg heads this initiative involving geneticists from across the country.

parent or sibling, and the age at which that relative developed AD. If a parent develops AD in his early sixties, the child has a higher risk than if the onset were in the parent's eighties. Studies also suggest that having more than one first-degree relative with Alzheimer's disease increases the risk.

More specifically, population studies suggest that when no family history of AD is present, there is approximately a 10 percent lifetime risk of developing the disease, and a family history of AD in close relatives can elevate one's lifetime risk to around 20 percent.

Dr. Schellenberg hypothesizes that a person who gets AD in his sixties may have more susceptibility genes than a person in his eighties. "If you had ten or fifteen individual genes that produced harmful proteins, you might get Alzheimer's disease quite a bit earlier. Those are the kind of genetic changes we're trying to find. But I have to admit it's highly unlikely that genes alone influence whether you get the disease. There is almost certainly a combination of genes and something in the environment—such as diet, lifestyle, or head trauma—that we don't yet understand."

But if your parent develops Alzheimer's in the early eighties, "like my dad did, that's typical. As people grow old, everyone's risk gets pretty high. As a geneticist, I think my father didn't have many susceptibility genes. Therefore, I probably do not have that many. I'm not that worried about my risk."

Eventually, geneticists may be able to create personalized genetic risk profiles to help predict who might develop AD. However, as Dr. Schellenberg says, and as most scientists agree, he's not in favor of genetic testing at our current state of knowledge. "It's important to know your risk if you can do something about it. Right now, even if we could predict who is going to get Alzheimer's disease when they're fifty, there is nothing we can do. I think we'll be there soon, but we're not there yet. I'm optimistic now that we're going to start coming up with good therapies in the next five or ten years."

A Susceptible Family

Dr. Richard Mayeux, a neurologist at Columbia University whose primary focus is genetics, is the lead researcher for the NIA's Alzheimer's Disease Genetics Initiative. He has conducted some of the most important genetic population studies, and he is currently studying an unusual family in a small town in rural Tennessee, the Nanney-Felt family. Usually, the study of very large numbers of individuals is required to isolate susceptibility genes. The Nanney-Felt family, however, presents a special case that Dr. Mayeux believes may be revealing in its own right, since they have such a high incidence of late-onset AD.

When Dr. Mayeux finds a family whose traits suggest that it is expressing a gene very strongly, he tries to find out everything he can about the family. In the case of a large family, where many individuals are affected by the disease in question, zeroing in on the genetics of a single family can yield useful scientific leads and insight into disease mechanisms.

The Nanney-Felts are one of the unusual families in which a susceptibility gene for late-onset Alzheimer's seems to be expressed very strongly among the members. The family traces the presence of AD back to a great-grandfather and his daughter, both of whom they believe showed signs of AD. The daughter had seven children, and, incredibly, all of them developed late-onset Alzheimer's disease in their mid-seventies. Some of their offspring are now showing early signs of the disease. The family became involved in the Alzheimer's Disease Genetics Initiative because of their concern for the fate of current and future generations.

Dr. Mayeux is studying their family tree as far back and as comprehensively as possible, collecting DNA samples from as many living members as he can track down, and following these family members over time. "We can start to trace a pattern," he says, "and it's quite possible that this family will have a unique susceptibility gene." He adds that locating such a gene would contribute yet another piece to the puzzle that is Alzheimer's disease.

7

LINKING ALZHEIMER'S DISEASE
AND VASCULAR DISEASE

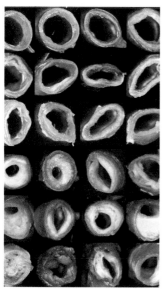

An extensive, intricate system of arteries and smaller capillaries brings a constant flow of oxygen and nutrients to every neuron in the brain. Consider that although the brain comprises only 2 percent of the body's mass, it uses 20 percent of the body's blood supply! The brain's vascular system is 400 miles long, with 400 billion capillaries. It is vital for brain health that these channels remain open.

Vascular conditions such as heart disease, high blood pressure, high cholesterol, and type 2 diabetes can damage and block the blood vessels throughout the body, including the brain. (Compare the normal arteries on top of the photograph on the previous page to the narrowed ones at the bottom, taken from major vessels that led to the brains of people who died with AD.) Vascular dementia, widely considered the second-most-common type of dementia, can result when massive strokes, or a series of small strokes, damage the brain. In addition, there may also be an association between vascular disease and AD.

Possible connections have been examined over time in population studies. Scientists also have conducted many studies in animals to confirm the associations and tease out their possible causes. Clinical trials are now under way in humans to test whether actions that reduce vascular disease risk factors may also reduce AD risk.

This chapter highlights some of the important research into possible associations between AD and vascular disease. Because vascular diseases are so common, this line of research is critical. Dr. Thomas Beach, a neuropathologist at Sun Health Research Institute, describes its significance, "The great potential of the vascular hypothesis in Alzheimer's disease is that we may be able to replicate the success that scientists in cardiovascular disease have had in preventing heart attacks and strokes. It's always more difficult to cure a disease once it's happened than to prevent it." Beach notes that medical science has had great success in preventing heart attacks and preventing strokes with the use of cholesterol-lowering medication and blood-pressure-lowering medication. The great potential, he says, is that if atherosclerotic vascular disease contributes even in part to Alzheimer's disease, we may be able to prevent it, to some extent, with drugs that are already tested and available.

Vascular Injury

Dr. Charles DeCarli, a neurologist at the University of California Davis Medical School, is studying the many ways that vascular disease injures the brain. "Twenty years ago, when researchers talked about diseases that affect the blood vessels of the brain, they were referring to strokes." With MRIs and other sensitive brain imaging tools, researchers can now visualize earlier stages of vascular disease in the brain. "We've moved from stroke to so-called silent strokes (strokes without symptoms), to small strokes called lacunae, to a type of very early injury called white matter hyperintensities. This has changed how we think about the ways vascular disease injures the brain."

When large blood vessels in the brain are completely blocked, a stroke occurs, significantly damaging an area of the brain. But earlier, less dramatic blockages can also damage the brain. Dr. DeCarli calls strokes "the tip of the iceberg of cerebrovascular disease." Some smaller vessels of the brain can become blocked, causing damage that produces no immediately discernible symptoms. These silent strokes may occur in as many as one in four people over the age of seventy-five. Other researchers have found that silent strokes double the risk of dementia, and that this kind of cerebrovascular disease intensifies the severity of AD.

Dr. DeCarli is also studying how vascular disease can harm neurons by damaging the axons. As we've seen, neurons communicate with each other by sending signals down the axon of one neuron and across the synapse to be received by the dendrite of a neighboring neuron. In order to better carry an electrical charge, the axon is insulated along its length by myelin, a fatty sheath produced by one of the brain's supporting cell types. By depriving it of blood and nutrients, vascular disease can damage the myelin. When this happens, the electrical impulse cannot travel as efficiently along the axon, and the neuron may not be able to send its signal to the neighboring cell. When neurons stop communicating, cognitive and other problems occur.

Dr. Charles DeCarli

▼

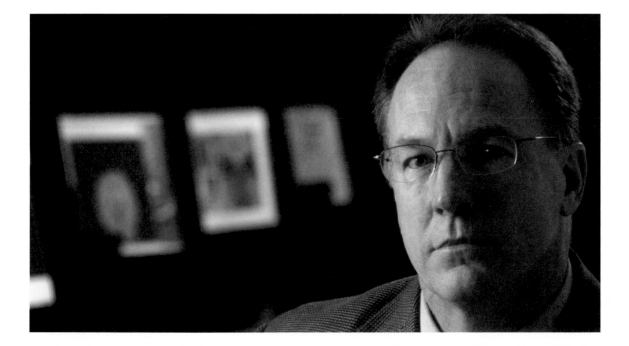

The Framingham Heart Study

Alzheimer's disease researchers are benefiting from decades of research on heart disease. The Framingham Heart Study is a prime example of this collaboration. In 1948, scientists funded by the National Heart, Lung, and Blood Institute came to the small city of Framingham, Massachusetts, to begin a long-term investigation of the physical and environmental factors that influence the development of heart disease. Two-thirds of the adults between the ages of thirty and sixty volunteered. In 1972, Framingham Heart Study scientists began following the children of the original group. In 2005, grandchildren joined the study.

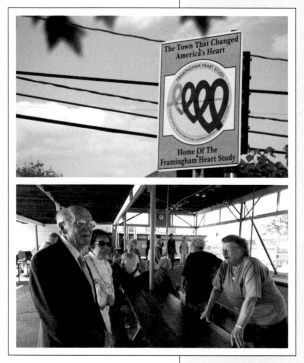

Dr. Richard Hodes explained that other National Institutes of Health institutes, including the National Institute on Aging, which he directs, have conducted a variety of "add-on studies" with this population. "This has allowed us to use all of the information gathered in this enormously important group, and to bring it to bear on a better understanding of the risk and protective factors that are relevant to dementia and Alzheimer's disease."

In 1999, Dr. Charles DeCarli joined the study of cognitive changes in dementia in the Framingham participants that is headed by Dr. Phil Wolf. He is using MRI imaging to examine how vascular disease may affect the size and shape of structures in the brain, possibly predisposing an individual to AD or other dementias. Because of the Framingham database, "We have forty to fifty years of blood pressure, cholesterol, blood sugar, and genetic information for each person, and have taken it into account when we've imaged how the shape of the brain changes in later life."

▲

Two volunteers (on left side of the table)—a lawyer who retired at the age of 93 and his wife—remain physically and cognitively active and engaged in their community

Dr. DeCarli and his team have refined MRI techniques to create a visual image of injured myelin around the axons. Damage shows up as bright white areas on a scan—what are called hyperintensities. "We're beginning to see evidence that if the axon is hurt by vascular disease, the whole nerve cell may die."

Vascular Disease and Alzheimer's Disease

Both vascular disease and Alzheimer's disease cause problems with thinking and memory and the death of brain tissue, although by different processes. However, as many as half of all brain autopsies conducted on people with AD reveal lesions characteristic of Alzheimer's disease as well as vascular lesions.

Researchers in many labs are still trying to understand the connection between the two conditions. There is, however, evidence already that both can exist independently in the same person. "Two injuries are worse than one," Dr. DeCarli said. "You're not going to do as well if you have both of those disease processes."

Using sophisticated MRI technology that provides highly accurate pictures of the shape and volume of brain structures, Dr. DeCarli is comparing the impact of the two disorders on the brain. He is focusing on the hippocampal formation, where very early indications of AD show themselves. If imaging shows that the hippocampus has shrunk, that suggests AD. If the effects of vascular disease are visible in other regions of the brain but the hippocampus looks normal, the person's thinking problems are more likely a result of vascular dementia. If Dr. DeCarli sees both, he reasons that both disease processes are occurring simultaneously.

As a researcher who also takes care of patients, Dr. DeCarli has treated people whom he suspects have both vascular dementia and Alzheimer's disease. Treatments exist for the vascular diseases that, when untreated, can lead to dementia, and Dr. DeCarli emphasizes they should be used when vascular disease is also present in a person with AD.

If a person with Alzheimer's disease also has hypertension, the doctor should treat it, he says. If she has diabetes, the doctor should treat the diabetes along with the Alzheimer's. And, Dr. DeCarli says, treating both diseases is likely to yield a better outcome than treating one.

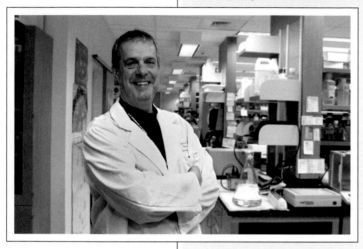

Dr. Berislav Zlokovic, a neuroscientist at the University of Rochester Medical School, is looking at ways that vascular disease may contribute to the buildup of beta-amyloid in the brain. Normally, blood carries excess beta-amyloid out of the brain to the liver and kidneys, which can dispose of it. In people with Alzheimer's disease, the removal system no longer functions properly.

Recently, Dr. Zlokovic and his research team have described a neurovascular hypothesis of AD that states that the faulty clearance of beta-amyloid across the blood-brain barrier, a diminished ability to develop new capillaries, and abnormal aging of the brain's blood vessel system can lead to chemical imbalances that damage the ability of nerve cells to communicate with each other. This hypothesis may help explain part of what happens in the brain as AD progresses. As with many of the other breakthroughs, these findings are also important because they suggest potential targets for drug development.

The Problem of Cholesterol

Cholesterol is essential for life. It is a component of cell membranes in mammals and is necessary for proper membrane function. Transported in the blood of all animals, cholesterol can come from the diet, can be recycled within the body through reabsorption, or can be produced "from scratch" by the liver. Cholesterol comprises about 25 percent of the brain's mass, and, in addition to being part of the cell membranes, it is a key component of myelin. However, too much cholesterol in the blood increases the risk of vascular disease. High blood cholesterol can lead to the buildup of plaques in the walls of blood vessels, restricting and possibly blocking the flow of blood; this condition is called atherosclerosis.

The association between high blood cholesterol and Alzheimer's disease is under intense investigation. One hypothesis is that the cholesterol-filled plaques in blood vessels contribute to Alzheimer's disease by restricting blood flow to the brain, damaging but not killing neurons. Scientists also speculate that cholesterol may be involved in the metabolism of beta-amyloid, though this process is not yet fully understood. Studies in animals have found that a high-cholesterol diet can increase beta-amyloid deposits in the hippocampus. Other animal studies show that when AD transgenic mice are given a statin (a cholesterol-lowering drug), both their blood cholesterol and their beta-amyloid levels decrease. Recent large clinical trials examining the effectiveness of statins in slowing the progression of AD in patients with mild to moderate AD did not show an effect. However, there are a number of clinical trials now examining whether earlier treatment with statins might delay the onset of AD in individuals with MCI or at risk for AD.

What's Good for the Heart Is Good for the Brain

Dr. DeCarli's research suggests that older people without vascular risk factors or evidence of vascular brain injury perform just like young people on cognitive tests. "If we could control vascular risk factors, maybe our brains could stay young, and we wouldn't have to experience the memory loss that is typical of aging," Dr. DeCarli suggested. "We know that Alzheimer's disease, which ten or twenty years ago was thought of as senility and a part of normal aging, is a pathological process. We need to take the next step and say the same is true of vascular disease." With that approach, we may prevent a lot of late-life cognitive impairment if we prevent vascular disease from accumulating. "We have medications that may turn back some of the vascular injury, but isn't it better to prevent that injury in the first place?" DeCarli says, proposing that exercise and lifestyle changes that reduce heart disease may prevent Alzheimer's disease as well.

"When we think about high blood pressure, when we think about diabetes, when we think about high cholesterol, we usually think about heart attacks." Lowering cholesterol is important for the heart, but it may be just as important for the brain, maybe even more important, according to DeCarli. Prevention is key. "Some heart damage can be repaired surgically, but not brain damage. A memory lost is never recovered."

As Dr. DeCarli indicated, we have prevention and treatment approaches for vascular disease, but people don't always follow them, or they begin too late. Half of people diagnosed with high blood pressure don't take their medications regularly. Many people who have had a stroke have not seen a doctor in years. There is danger here, because the longer vascular disease goes untreated, the more it damages the whole body, including the brain.

The damage often begins when people are in their thirties and forties. The early changes that increase the risk of vascular disease have few or no symptoms: high blood pressure, high blood cholesterol, and problems with insulin control, so it often goes undetected in the early stage unless a person has regular checkups and blood tests.

"People can make changes in exercise, diet, blood pressure, smoking, and cholesterol levels," Dr. DeCarli explained. "They can see their doctors regularly to check blood pressure, blood sugar, and cholesterol and to get conditions like high blood pressure, heart disease, and diabetes diagnosed early. They can control obesity and carefully manage their diabetes. All these steps will protect the blood vessels so they continue to deliver blood to the brain." If we take care of our bodies now, he suggests, our bodies might take care of our brains later.

Compared to fifty years ago, many more people can live vigorous, productive lives well into their eighties if they take care of themselves. Dr. DeCarli believes that people may be able to reach the age of eighty with no memory problems, if they've done everything they can to control their vascular risk factors. "I dream that the memory loss of old age will one day be history."

Atherosclerosis and Alzheimer's Disease

Dr. Thomas Beach runs the Banner Sun Health Research Institute brain bank in Sun City, Arizona. Dr. Beach sees and catalogues many samples of brain tissue that Sun City residents have donated to research after they die. "We have found that Alzheimer's disease patients are about two times more likely to have clogged blood vessels or severe atherosclerosis than people who are cognitively normal." The problem is particularly common in the blood vessels at the base of the brain.

Dr. Beach describes atherosclerosis as inflammation caused by cholesterol deposits on an artery wall. "The deposit is like a little sore, an open wound." The body's white blood cells target the inflammation and try to repair it. The white blood cells and other material released in the healing process slip into the lining of the artery, where they accumulate and create more inflammation. Additionally, a fibrous material forms and then hardens within the artery lining. This plaque builds up over time and blocks the flow of blood. "It's shocking the extent to which some of these brain arteries are plugged up by yellowish cholesterol deposits. In some of the

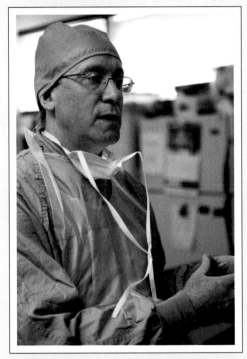

arteries, the area for the blood to flow through is extremely small or nonexistent.

"We think that there is definitely some kind of relationship between atherosclerotic vascular disease and Alzheimer's disease. We don't know if it's causative or coincidental. If it is causative, we don't understand the mechanism by which atherosclerosis influences Alzheimer's disease. Inflammation may be behind both." Dr. Beach hypothesizes that certain molecules may start an inflammatory process in brain capillaries. Once this happens, the brain capillaries do not function as well, which, as Dr. Zlokovic described, may reduce the ability to deliver excess beta-amyloid from the brain to the liver and kidneys for disposal.

"Excess beta-amyloid should cross the capillary wall into the bloodstream. If the capillaries aren't doing their job because of inflammation, they may not be getting rid of beta-amyloid the way they should. The beta-amyloid can accumulate in the brain as amyloid plaques." Dr. Beach agrees with other researchers that the drugs and lifestyle changes that have successfully addressed vascular disease may well prove valuable in the prevention of Alzheimer's disease.

8

ASSOCIATING ALZHEIMER'S DISEASE WITH INSULIN RESISTANCE AND DIABETES

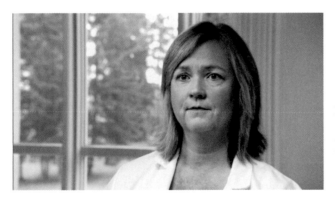

Scientists are increasingly recognizing that, even though Alzheimer's disease is a brain disease, conditions that affect the rest of the body may also influence the pathways that may lead to it. As we've seen, a growing collection of research, including the work of **Dr. Suzanne Craft,** suggests that the risk of cognitive decline and AD may increase with vascular diseases such as heart disease and the related conditions of high blood cholesterol and high blood pressure. The metabolic disease called diabetes also affects the vascular system and is another area of intense interest among AD researchers. Epidemiological studies have shown that people with diabetes have an increased risk of cognitive problems, including MCI and AD, as they age. This has inspired a number of experimental studies exploring the possible connections between diabetes and AD.

Dr. Suzanne Craft, a professor of psychiatry and behavioral science at the VA Puget Sound and the University of Washington School of Medicine and a leading researcher in this area, hypothesizes that insulin resistance, a condition that precedes and characterizes type 2 diabetes, plays a significant role in the AD process. "For a long time, this idea was out of the mainstream," she observed. Today, insulin resistance is being studied as a possible pathway to AD.

Insulin resistance is a key component of metabolic syndrome, a group of vascular and metabolic abnormalities, which is associated with accelerated decline in cognitive abilities during aging. The elements of metabolic syndrome include obesity (especially around the waist), high triglyceride levels, low HDL ("good" blood cholesterol) levels, high blood pressure, and insulin resistance. Epidemiological studies suggest that each of these vascular and metabolic abnormalities is associated with an elevated risk of AD.

Diabetes and Insulin Resistance

Diabetes is a chronic metabolic disorder in which the body doesn't produce or properly use insulin, a hormone that is made in the pancreas and is essential for the healthy functioning of all cells in the body. After a meal, the digestive system breaks most food down into glucose, a form of sugar that travels in the bloodstream throughout the body and powers cellular activity. In the blood and in the brain, insulin helps glucose enter cells. As glucose levels rise in the blood after a meal, the pancreas releases insulin to help cells take in and use the glucose. Insulin released by the pancreas after a meal and throughout the day is transported into the brain, where it has important effects on brain function.

About 5–10 percent of people with diabetes have type 1 diabetes, an autoimmune disease that attacks the pancreas so that it can no longer make insulin. By far the more common form of diabetes is type 2, a condition in which the pancreas makes enough insulin but the cells do not respond properly to it—a condition called insulin resistance.

In insulin resistance, the pancreas works overtime to make more insulin to help glucose enter cells, so insulin levels rise in the blood. No matter how much insulin the pancreas produces, it can't control glucose levels, and glucose builds up in the blood, creating high blood glucose levels. Many people with insulin resistance have high levels of both glucose and insulin in their blood. When a certain threshold is crossed, a person will be diagnosed with type 2 diabetes.

Risk factors for insulin resistance and type 2 diabetes are obesity (particularly excess fat at the waist), lack of exercise, increased age, and genetic factors. Many people with type 2 diabetes have no symptoms at first. When symptoms begin to emerge, they can include infections, vision problems, nerve damage, extreme thirst, and fatigue. Over time, diabetes damages the heart, blood vessels, eyes, kidneys, and nerves. These complications can be reduced by managing blood glucose levels through weight control, diet, exercise, medications, and, sometimes, the administration of insulin injections.

Type 2 diabetes affects almost one fifth of Americans over sixty. More than twenty-three million Americans have diabetes, including nearly six million who don't know they have it. Millions of others have insulin resistance. "With the increase in obesity, the lack of physical activity, and changes in our diet," Dr. Craft told us, "this is a rapidly growing condition."

Insulin in the Brain

Scientists have known for a long time that insulin is critical to the healthy functioning of the body's many types of cells. Like other cells in the body, neurons in the brain need glucose to fuel their activities. In fact, PET scans have revealed that when some parts of the brain are engaged in a demanding cognitive task, the neurons in that area metabolize a great deal of glucose.

Within minutes of a meal, insulin is sent to the brain to help neurons absorb and use glucose. Smaller increases in insulin also occur throughout the day, likely in response to neural signals. Dr. Craft explained, "In the brain, insulin has a number of roles to play. It promotes glucose uptake in the neurons of the hippocampal formation and the frontal lobes," areas that are involved in memory. Insulin also strengthens the synaptic connections between brain cells, helping to form new memories. In addition, insulin regulates the neurotransmitter acetylcholine, which plays an important role in learning and memory. Finally, insulin is involved in blood vessel formation and function. Dr. Craft speculated that the many links between eating, insulin, and memory could have evolved for survival reasons. "It was important to remember where you got the food and if the food was good or made you sick. From an evolutionary perspective, the linkage of eating and memory is very close."

Dr. Craft is studying the relationship between insulin and glucose in people with Alzheimer's disease. Her research was first inspired by epidemiological data suggesting that people with diabetes and insulin resistance have an increased risk of cognitive problems, including MCI and AD, as they grow old. She wondered whether insulin resistance reduces the ability of insulin to get into the brain, leaving the brain without enough for normal functioning.

She and her team began a series of human studies to explore the relationships among glucose and insulin levels in the brain, memory performance, and AD pathology. PET scans had shown that people with Alzheimer's disease metabolize less glucose in specific areas of their brains. Dr. Craft wanted to know if there were ways to raise the level of glucose in the brains of people with AD. She began with a small-scale test in which she asked research volunteers to consume a high-glucose drink and then take a short-term memory test.

Memory performance increased temporarily, but so did insulin levels. This made sense, because a rise in blood glucose signals the pancreas to produce more insulin. "We realized that every time we raised glucose, we were also raising insulin. And we noticed that the people with higher insulin levels showed the most memory benefit. We wondered if the insulin was enhancing memory, not just the glucose." In a follow-up study, they raised glucose levels, but gave a medication that stopped insulin from being secreted. They found that without insulin the memory improvement did not occur.

From these early studies, Dr. Craft and her team made two observations: Research volunteers with AD experienced a much higher increase in insulin from the glucose intake than did volunteers without AD, and insulin had to be present for the glucose to help improve memory.

Next, the researchers isolated insulin's effect by raising insulin through an intravenous infusion without raising glucose levels. Memory improved, leading Dr. Craft and her team to conclude that the difference in memory performance is likely the result of increased levels of insulin, not glucose.

The team then gave normal older adult volunteers a larger dose of insulin, enough to mimic the high levels that occur when a person has insulin resistance. After this infusion, the team analyzed the spinal fluid, which had been obtained through lumbar punctures, for levels of proteins like beta-amyloid. The researchers were "quite surprised" to see a rapid increase in beta-amyloid levels following the administration of higher levels of insulin. Dr. Craft said. "This was especially pronounced in older adults. Their beta-amyloid increased 25 percent." Dr. Craft's study showed that high insulin levels might affect the amount of beta-amyloid in the spinal fluid. "As far as I know, this was the first demonstration in humans that changes in the levels of insulin in the blood can result in changes in beta-amyloid."

In a different study, which is currently ongoing, she next induced temporary insulin resistance through a high-fat/high-sugar diet to study its effects on beta-amyloid and blood cholesterol. She asked one group of research volunteers to follow the high-fat/high-sugar diet for four weeks, and another group to follow a low-fat/low-sugar diet. The preliminary results show that, in just a month, the participants on the high-fat/high-sugar diet had changes in beta-amyloid in the spinal fluid that may adversely impact its clearance from the brain and significant increases in LDL cholesterol ("bad" blood cholesterol). Those on the low-fat/low-sugar diet had improved beta-amyloid, insulin, and cholesterol profiles. Dr. Craft speculated that the temporary insulin resistance induced by the high-fat/high-sugar diet interfered with the clearance of beta-amyloid, perhaps by affecting the enzyme in the liver that normally clears beta-amyloid from the bloodstream. (We will return to this study and others related to diet in Chapter 11.)

Based on this series of studies, Dr. Craft hypothesized that insulin resistance (with high levels of insulin in the body) paradoxically leads to lower-than-normal levels of insulin in the brain, which results in memory problems. The studies suggest that introducing more insulin to the brain might restore the proper balance of insulin and improve memory. However, more insulin in the rest of the body would be harmful, because it would increase insulin resistance and beta-amyloid levels.

The Studies of Nasal Insulin to Fight Forgetfulness (SNIFF)

In response to this observation, Dr. Craft devised a study that raised the level of insulin in the brain but not in the rest of the body. She decided to use a nebulizer, a device that administers medicine in the form of a mist, to deliver insulin directly to the upper sinuses. From there, the molecules of insulin could enter the brain via a direct pathway that bypasses the bloodstream—thereby avoiding both the difficulty of passing through the blood-brain barrier and the problem of raising insulin levels in the body. In animal studies of this nasal spray technique, Dr. Craft pointed out, peptides similar to insulin follow direct pathways to the brain and reach the hippocampus, a brain region important in learning and memory, in fifteen to thirty minutes.

Dr. Craft tested whether delivering insulin this way affected memory in people with Alzheimer's disease. Adults with AD had better memory for stories and lists after receiving a single dose of intranasal insulin. In a separate study, the research team administered insulin to people with early-onset AD twice a day for three weeks; the patients also had success retaining the details of a story, as well as paying attention to information when presented with a distraction.

These results led to a larger clinical trial, now in progress, called the SNIFF 120 trial, an acronym for the Study of Nasal Insulin to

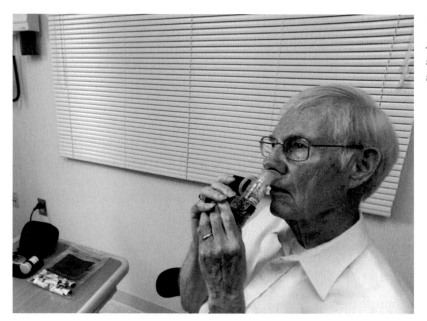

A volunteer in Dr. Craft's SNIFF study practices using a nebulizer to administer insulin to his brain.

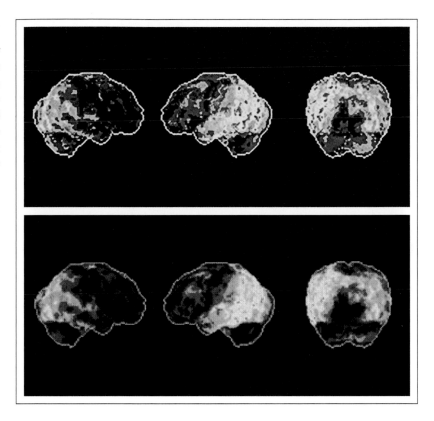

These scans show three views of the brain of a person with AD before intranasal insulin treatment (above) and four months later (below). Improved glucose metabolism is shown by more and larger areas of dark blue, and fewer and smaller areas of red, orange, and yellow.

Fight Forgetfulness. Study participants receive insulin via a nasal spray twice a day for four months. The trial is examining the effects of insulin delivered in this way on cognitive function in people with amnestic MCI or AD, including the ability to carry out daily activities. In addition, "We are measuring glucose metabolism in their brains using PET scans before and after the treatment period. We're measuring beta-amyloid in their spinal fluid before and after treatment, as well as their cognitive function. Quantifying the change in glucose metabolism will allow us to determine if that predicts the degree of cognitive improvement. That will help us understand a little bit better the mechanism underlying the potential cognitive improvement," Dr. Craft told us.

Through research like Dr. Craft's, we may discover that therapies that increase insulin in the brain or counteract insulin resistance may someday be used to help prevent or treat AD. In the meantime, strategies such as diet and exercise can lower the risk of insulin resistance and type 2 diabetes, and may reduce the risk of cognitive decline and AD.

Dr. Craft observed that neuroscientists tend to undervalue the impact of diseases originating in other parts of the body, while scientists studying other diseases have little idea of the impact those diseases could have on the brain. She and others are enthusiastic about the gains that may come from continued collaboration between AD research and diabetes research. She described an air of excitement: "People are now starting to understand the critical interaction between the brain and the body and that many of the peptides and hormones produced in the body have very substantial roles to play in the brain. I think we're at the beginning of a very exciting era in which we're going to be able to start putting together these systems to understand Alzheimer's disease, which is clearly a disease of the entire organism, not just of the brain. We're happy to be part of the forefront of bringing this into reality."

9

LEARNING ABOUT
THE ROLE OF INFLAMMATION

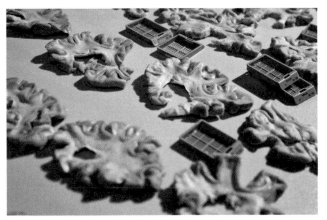

By attacking and ridding the body of injured tissue, infectious agents, and potentially toxic foreign matter, inflammatory mechanisms represent one of the immune system's first lines of defense. Although these mechanisms can be brought into play nearly anywhere in the body, for many years it was thought that immune and inflammatory cells were kept completely out of the brain by the blood-brain barrier. Lacking its own immune or inflammatory cells, the brain was therefore considered to be "immunologically privileged" and incapable of mounting any kind of inflammatory response on its own. This idea now turns out to be wrong on both counts. Despite some hindrance by the blood-brain barrier, immune and inflammatory cells can gain access to the brain, and the brain is now known to contain an intrinsic cell type that can launch a nearly full repertoire of inflammatory responses.

Since the 1920s, in fact, scientists have recognized that microglia, specialized scavenger cells that respond to brain lesions, exist in the brain, but the possibility that microglia could play an inflammatory role in brain disorders was not well recognized until the mid-1980s. Although we now know that microglia can mediate inflammatory responses in many neurologic conditions, including Parkinson's disease, Lou Gehrig's disease (ALS), and HIV/AIDS dementia, the original discovery was made in the context of Alzheimer's disease. Today, researchers universally agree that inflammation does occur in the brain, and they are trying to discover whether, when unchecked, it plays a role in the development and progression of Alzheimer's disease. Could inflammation prove to be yet another possible pathway to Alzheimer's disease?

Dr. Joe Rogers, a genial, dynamic proponent of the role of inflammation in Alzheimer's disease and several other neurologic disorders,

Dr. Joe Rogers

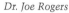

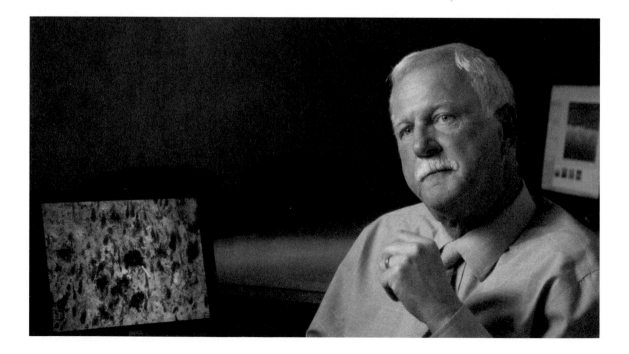

has been investigating inflammatory and immune responses to beta-amyloid plaques for more than two decades. He is one of a group of scientists credited with the discovery that the brain's immune system recognizes beta-amyloid plaques as potentially toxic, "foreign" matter and launches an immune response to try to remove it. He is also the founder of the Banner Sun Health Research Institute, which is a partner in the Arizona Alzheimer's Consortium and one of the National Institute on Aging's network of twenty-nine Alzheimer's Disease Centers.

Brain Inflammation

In the body, inflammatory responses usually occur as a local reaction. To heal a cut or a scrape, for example, special cells are dispatched quickly to attack bacteria or foreign matter. However, when triggered inappropriately or regulated poorly, inflammatory responses can become chronic and can damage tissues and organs that otherwise are healthy. Rheumatoid arthritis, for example, is a disease in which the body's immune system mistakenly attacks its own tissues, causing pain, swelling, and joint deterioration.

Inflammation is generally beneficial—one of the main ways the body has to heal itself and expel foreign intruders—but its defensive measures can cause collateral damage. Dr. Rogers explained, "Inflammation is always a two-edged sword. It's a complex set of body processes that identify, attack, and remove foreign invaders from the body. Some components of inflammation are highly destructive—among the most toxic mechanisms in the body. When they target a bacterium that's causing an infection, that's a very good thing." However, during the immune system's natural process of destroying cells that it recognizes as foreign, the inflammatory response can sometimes damage normal tissue, as well. Dr. Rogers and other scientists have shown that, in Alzheimer's disease, neurons in the parts of the brain most intimately connected with memory and cognition may be inadvertently destroyed when the brain's microglia target and attempt to remove beta-amyloid deposits.

Early Observations

Beta-amyloid plaques are hard to break up, and, in the laboratory, scientists must use extremely strong acids to dissolve them if they're to be studied. When Dr. Rogers first saw these plaques through the microscope lens many years ago, their dense aggregation, profusion, and foreign, abnormal appearance struck him as having the potential to stimulate inflammation. "It looked as if someone had thrown a handful of dirt into the patient's brain." When the immune system detects something abnormal and foreign such as dirt in a cut, it launches an inflammatory attack. Why wouldn't the presence of these sticky plaques in the brain trigger a similarly strong reaction?

To test his hunch, Dr. Rogers stained a section of brain tissue from a person who had died with Alzheimer's disease using a special marker that only binds to cells involved in an active inflammatory response. He saw thousands of cells decorated with that marker, which indicated many sites of active inflammation. This suggested that an inflammatory response might well be occurring in the Alzheimer's brain. Significantly, the inflammatory activity was happening in areas of the brain involved in higher mental functions such as decision-making and memory—precisely the areas and functions that are hard hit by Alzheimer's disease. When he used the same marker in brain areas responsible for motor function, he found no inflammatory cells. Nor did he find significant inflammation in brain tissue from healthy elderly people.

In these initial studies, Dr. Rogers used slices of brain tissue from autopsies, so he couldn't see the cells in action. "We wanted to look at inflammation in living cells, where we could observe inflammatory changes occurring and understand how they worked. We're very fortunate to be able to do that here at Banner Sun Health Research Institute. Even after someone dies, many cells in the body remain alive for anywhere from a few minutes to a few hours. Because we're willing to get up in the middle of the night, if necessary, to do the autopsies, we're often able to get living cells out of the brains of people who've volunteered to be in our tissue bank after they die. We can keep the cells going using a special technique called tissue culture. With the methods we've developed, scientists now have living microglia from Alzheimer's and normal brains with which to do experiments."

Microglia and Beta-Amyloid

When Dr. Rogers examined the stained clusters surrounding the beta-amyloid, he saw that these cells had wrapped themselves all around the plaques. "At first, I didn't know what the cells were. I had never seen anything like them." He later realized that they were microglia, the specialized scavenger cells that rid the brain of damaged neurons and other cellular debris.

Microglia were able to engulf and remove beta-amyloid in tissue cultures. "In the dishes where we grew these cells, we first put down a tiny spot of beta-amyloid to mimic the plaques in the brain of a person with Alzheimer's disease. We then seeded the dishes with living microglia from people who had had Alzheimer's disease. At first, the microglia were randomly distributed. Over a few days, they migrated to the margins of the beta-amyloid spot. In a few more days, the microglia completely covered the spot. They seemed to attack the beta-amyloid and eat it. The stain we had used for the beta-amyloid was brown, and we noticed that the microglia cells turned brown, too, from clumps of beta-amyloid they had ingested." These findings suggested that microglia may do some good by removing beta-amyloid, and they served as some of the inspiration behind the work of Dr. Dale Schenk. A researcher at Elan Pharmaceuticals, Dr. Schenk has developed a possible vaccine against amyloid plaques. (We will cover this in Chap-

High-power microscopic view of microglia (isolated spots), the brain's scavenger inflammatory response cells, devouring a beta-amyloid plaque (surrounding mass).

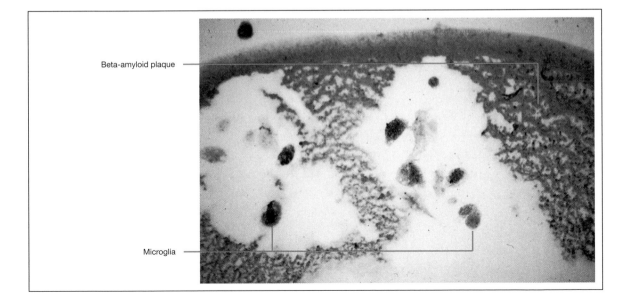

Beta-amyloid plaque

Microglia

ter 12.) If we can provoke and enhance the brain's inflammatory response against beta-amyloid, Dr. Schenk postulated, perhaps we can harness the strength of the body's own immune system and recruit it in the fight against Alzheimer's pathology.

But the activity of microglia can also be destructive. Dr. Rogers and his team found that the beta-amyloid deposits, as well as parts of nearby nerve cells, were also covered with molecules called complement, a highly destructive weapon in the immune system's arsenal. Complement not only acts as a beacon to microglia, signaling them to attack the plaques, but it also can damage or destroy healthy bystander cells. One of the complement components, for example, creates a hole in the outer covering of cells. "The cells spring a leak," Dr. Rogers explained. "If a bacterium springs a leak, it's a good thing because you just killed it. But if a healthy nerve cell gets caught up in the process of removing something like beta-amyloid, it's not good at all."

Anti-Inflammatory Drugs

Besides the work being done to develop drugs that would exploit the positive, destructive effects of the brain's inflammatory response to beta-amyloid, researchers are also looking into drugs that might minimize the negative aspects of the chronic inflammation that may be present in the plaque-ridden Alzheimer's brain. Interestingly, epidemiological studies have associated long-term use of nonsteroidal anti-inflammatory drugs (NSAIDs), such as naproxen or ibuprofen, with a decreased risk of Alzheimer's disease. In the early stages of his research on inflammation, Dr. Rogers conducted one such study with Dr. Patrick McGeer of the University of British Columbia. They surveyed people who had a primary diagnosis of arthritis and took anti-inflammatory drugs regularly. They compared this population to people the same age with other diagnoses. "We found that the people with arthritis, who presumably had been taking NSAIDs for years, were four to five times less likely to develop symptoms of Alzheimer's disease."

Today, in fact, some two dozen studies of NSAID use in normal middle-aged and elderly people have confirmed Dr. Rogers's and Dr. McGeer's original findings. Unfortunately, however, whether NSAIDs might influence the active disease process and, if so, how still remains unclear. Laboratory and animal research suggests that some NSAIDs may decrease the production of beta-amyloid, creating a protective pathway. Scientists have conducted studies in cell cultures and AD transgenic mice to assess the effects of many NSAIDs on beta-amyloid production, and they have found that a number of common NSAIDs reduced beta-amyloid levels in mice and in cell cultures.

To date, however, clinical trials to explore this relationship further and determine whether anti-inflammatory drugs might help slow the progression of Alzheimer's disease have not demonstrated any benefit. Nevertheless, scientists are still exploring ways to test whether anti-inflammatory drugs could affect the development or progression of the disorder. Dr. Rogers, who believes that anti-inflammatory drugs may ultimately prove useful against Alzheimer's disease, emphasizes that "we need to run more larger-scale clinical trials, particularly prevention trials, with people like you and me to make sure that the risk is worth the potential benefit. That has not been done—and, until it has, I can't recommend taking NSAIDs to ward off Alzheimer's disease to anyone."

SUN CITY BRAIN BANK

Alzheimer's disease researchers perform many experiments on brain tissue. They rely on healthy and diseased brain tissues that were generously donated to AD research by people around the country to be used after death. The support of the retirement community of Sun City, Arizona, has been especially inspiring. Many Sun City residents have agreed to participate in AD studies at the Banner Sun Health Research Institute.

"When I first came to the area in 1986," Dr. Rogers told us, "there were no buildings, equipment, money, or staff. But this was the ideal place to do research in Alzheimer's disease. All the patients are here! Some of the greatest minds in Alzheimer's disease research may be in Cambridge, Massachusetts, but the people you need for research have long since moved to a warmer climate. We have spent all the years since cultivating a close relationship with the members of this community."

The massive retirement community does have a large pool of potential research participants. The area is home to around two hundred thousand people, and the average age is seventy-two; an older population includes more people at risk of

Alzheimer's disease than in the general population because risk increases with age. Moreover, they live near Dr. Rogers's research facility, making conducting clinical studies efficient.

Just as important, though, is the spirit of volunteerism in the community. The all-volunteer Sun City Prides clean the streets, the Sun City Posse serves as the town's law enforcement, and residents eagerly sign up for clinical trials and volunteer at the Banner Sun Health Research Institute. "Of our staff of one hundred at the research institute, about twenty-three are unpaid volunteers from the community, including three retired PhD chemists. Two of them have published more papers in their retirement with us than they did as professors at the university. The retired chief of staff at the hospital across the street now works in our clinical center. Retired librarians keep our journals, and clerical people help with our books."

Many residents have donated their brains upon death. The tissue bank has recruited 2 percent of the community's population by word of mouth and through the unique tours that Dr. Rogers has instituted at the center, which allow the community to see what goes on in the laboratories. There are no financial inducements and no advertising. "Almost all the people who are enrolled in the tissue bank have heard me speak at the Rotary Club, the VFW, the Catholic Women's Club, or the Lutheran Men's

Edith Brozka, 86, a volunteer at the Banner Sun Health Research Institute, proudly gives a tour of the lab.

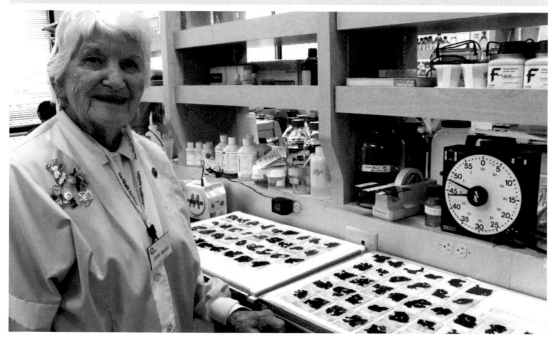

Club. People have told me, 'Joe, I'm really happy for you to take my brain after I die. I want to do something good with it, and you've given me this opportunity.'"

Here, too, proximity to the center is an advantage. When a person dies, the loss of oxygen and nutrients causes brain tissue to deteriorate rapidly. In the 1980s, neuroscientist Dr. Allen Roses and his team at Duke University devised a system with local pathologists to monitor people who had agreed to donate their brains when they were close to death. Within two hours of a death, the pathologists were able to process the brain tissue and send it to Dr. Roses. Dr. Rogers and other scientists subsequently adopted this rapid autopsy procedure so that they could study brain biochemistry in tissue that is still similar to what it was when the patient was alive, and before degrading enzymes in the brain began to break it down.

This was a big step forward, as Dr. Thomas Beach, the neuropathologist who runs the Banner Sun Health Research Institute brain bank, explained. "We're all really just a bag of chemical reactions. We're full of water, and there are millions of chemical reactions going on. That is what makes us living, that is what makes us function. The longer after death that we look, the more the molecules have changed to something else from what they were during life. So clearly, if we want to understand the chemistry of disease, which is the chemistry of life, we want to freeze that chemistry as soon as we can after death. It was a great idea for Dr. Rogers to start the brain bank twenty years ago. Not only just to start it, but to emphasize the rapid autopsy."

Once the brain has been removed during autopsy, the lab examines it to determine if it contains an abundance of beta-amyloid plaques. If that is the case, and

---

After autopsy, brain slices are prepared for freezing.

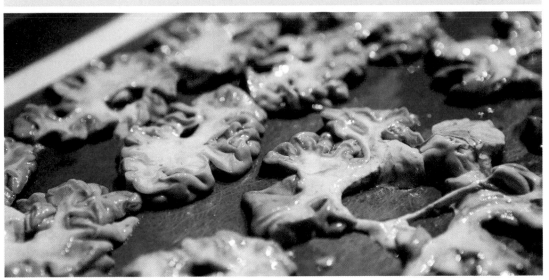

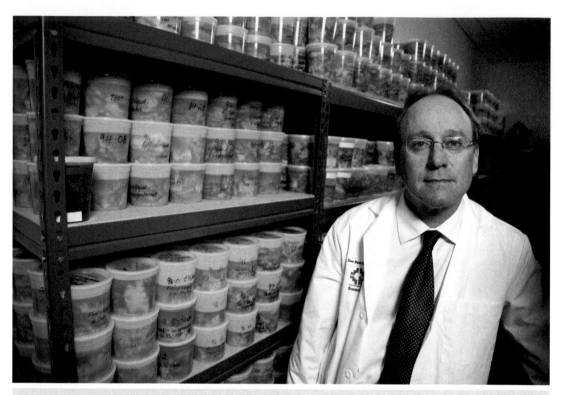

Dr. Thomas Beach at the brain bank.

---

the person has neurofibrillary tangles and was severely cognitively impaired during life, then the person can be confirmed to have had Alzheimer's disease.

After the team has taken the pieces of tissue needed to make the diagnosis under the microscope, they freeze half of the brain at minus 80 degrees Celsius (minus 112 degrees Fahrenheit). This is cold enough that the brain tissue will remain similar to how it was at death, for decades. Anytime a researcher asks for control tissue or tissue that shows signs of Alzheimer's disease, the lab can send it out. Such use is agreed to by the individuals and families that generously participate in the brain donation programs that are helping to advance AD research.

The tissue bank at Sun City has grown into a very large program. Dr. Rogers said, "I like to tell people from Sun City that even if the final experiment that gives us the answer to Alzheimer's disease is not done in Sun City, it's likely to be done on a Sun Citian, because tissue from our program goes out to the very best investigators all over the world, from the United States to Russia to Japan. We send it gladly to do our part."

IV

CHANGING THE OUTLOOK

Scientists have made many breakthrough discoveries about the way Alzheimer's disease begins and progresses. Researchers have made tremendous strides in understanding the major pathological characteristics of AD in the brain, beta-amyloid plaques and neurofibrillary tangles, though our knowledge is still incomplete. The work being done now revolves around attaining a more thorough picture of how all the events involved in the Alzheimer's disease process fit together, and how the complex processes at work in AD have ripple effects throughout the brain, from neuronal overexcitation and inflammation to synaptic dysfunction and hippocampal hyperactivation. All this research into basic science is important because it opens up a variety of possibilities for treatment and prevention.

Each time a scientist clarifies a new aspect of the disease process, he or she may have found another chance to modify or change that process. For example, once researchers identified the two enzymes that cleave the APP protein to form beta-amyloid peptides (which can clump together to form plaques in the brain), drugs to block those enzymes were developed, and now some are being tested in clinical trials. Many more drugs in clinical trials have come out of basic science findings that illuminate various steps along the disease process. As we uncover more about the disease process, even more drug targets are certain to be identified.

Another major advance has been the emerging consensus that the processes that culminate in AD are set in motion long before symptoms appear, and that the ability to identify people at a pre-symptomatic stage increases the chance of having a positive drug effect before cognitive decline becomes life-changing. The ability to define mild cognitive impairment (MCI) as an early stage in functional decline represents another step forward in accurately delineating the boundaries between normal and impaired cognition that can progress to AD. Improved tools for early diagnosis will help scientists test drugs on the right populations, ideally early in the disease process before symptoms begin.

Both basic science and drug development have benefited from the groundbreaking advances in imaging technologies that have occurred in the last few years. Imaging tools currently used in research have allowed scientists to see the pathologies of AD in living brains, shedding new light on many aspects of the disease process. Imaging is now also a key element of many clinical trials, making it possible to start correlating physical changes in the brain with alterations in thinking and memory abilities.

Scientists are singling out and studying many possible contributing causes of AD, including risk factors such as vascular disease, diabetes and insulin resistance, and inflammation, all of which in turn can be influenced by inherited susceptibility genes. These contributing factors also suggest ways to shift the outlook on AD, which is the focus of Part IV. While we cannot do anything about our individual genome and age, research is suggesting that some lifestyle factors that are within our control may be important. There is accumulating evidence to suggest that exercise, diet, and cognitive stimulation may make a difference to the aging brain, particularly when maintained over the course of a lifetime. Scientists have also begun to explore the therapeutic implications of studies that have associated AD with vascular disease and diabetes.

It's fitting that the final chapter of *The Alzheimer's Project: Momentum in Science* focuses on the development of drugs to treat or prevent AD. Many people wonder why it is taking so long to develop drugs that can help their loved ones or decrease their own risk. Their impatience is perfectly understandable. But AD is a complicated disease, and the process by which a safe, effective drug can be brought to market is a difficult one to traverse. Developing a new drug takes a lot of time, money, scientists trained in many different disciplines, and research volunteers—not to mention scientific brilliance and a lot of luck. Fortunately, in the world of AD drug development, many scientists and organizations are working very hard to develop drugs that will make a difference.

The search for drug treatments begins with basic science and may well end with a new outcome for millions of people. We can chart a new path toward the future for AD research by supporting continued basic scientific inquiry and the advances in drug development and therapeutic strategies that will come from it. In the final chapters of this book, we step inside the laboratories and learn about the clinical trials that are bringing that future ever closer.

In a little more than twenty years, the science has come to a point where the expectation is now that a treatment will definitely be found to slow or even prevent the disease. "Our only sorrow," Dr. Steven DeKosky said, "is that we can't do it instantly."

10

BUILDING COGNITIVE RESERVE

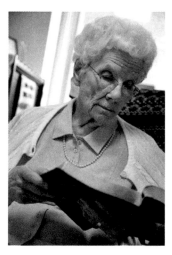

Now that PET scans with PiB can measure beta-amyloid levels in a living brain, studies have found that about 25 percent of seventy-year-olds have evidence of one pathology of Alzheimer's disease—beta-amyloid plaques—even without showing clinical symptoms of memory loss or cognitive decline. Although these people are cognitively normal, they have a substantial plaque load.

Dr. David Bennett, the director of the Rush Alzheimer's Disease Center at Rush University Medical Center in Chicago, has been researching this phenomenon. He is intrigued by cases like a ninety-year-old nun who had shown no decline in cognition but was found to have a substantial amount of beta-amyloid plaques upon autopsy. He wondered how she could have so much beta-amyloid in her brain but experience no evident memory loss.

Scientists do not doubt that beta-amyloid changes the brain, but researchers like Dr. Bennett are focusing on what enables some people's brains to withstand what could be damaging effects. Do they have a bigger brain, a better brain, a more efficient brain, or something else? In some cases, the brain may have some sort of "cognitive reserve," the ability to operate effectively even while damage is occurring.

Alzheimer's disease researchers such as Dr. Bennett are working to understand why some people have these brain reserves, which seem to protect them from presumed damage by beta-amyloid. What protective role might brain efficiency play? Could different personality traits make someone more or less susceptible to AD? How might early life experiences and lifelong behaviors affect the disease?

In particular, Dr. Bennett is studying the possible impact of behavior, lifestyle, and education on the aging brain. As the lead researcher on two major observational studies—the Rush Memory and Aging Project and the Religious Orders Study—he heads a team that is collect-

Dr. David Bennett

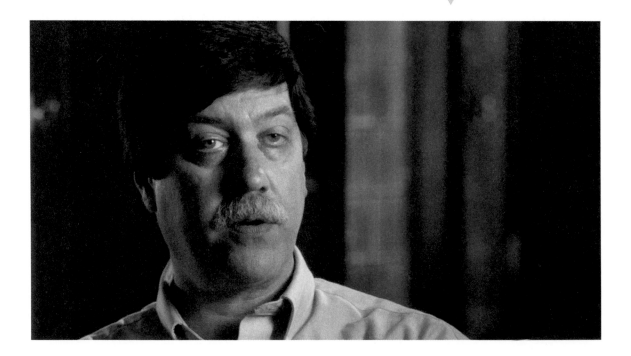

ing detailed family histories, socioeconomic data, and records of performance on cognitive exams over time from more than twenty-three hundred individuals and retirement home residents, including older Catholic nuns, priests, and brothers living in forty communities across the United States. All participants agree to donate their brains to science upon their death, and, to date, Dr. Bennett has collected more than seven hundred brains to study. A third of people enrolled in the study, including the nun described above, are found upon autopsy to have fully developed Alzheimer's disease plaque pathology without any obvious cognitive problems. He hypothesizes that cognitive reserve may be preventing these brains from expressing clinical signs of Alzheimer's disease.

Brain Efficiency

At one time, scientists believed that people with cognitive reserve had simply been born with bigger brains; that they had more neurons, so if some nerve cells died as a result of Alzheimer's disease or other disease processes, others were waiting to take over. This theory has been disproved—any connection between brain size and cognition is quite subtle.

Imaging studies have provided compelling evidence that brain efficiency, not size, underlies cognitive capacity. Brain scans show that a person learning a new task engages a great deal of the brain or has greater activity in a particular region. As the task becomes familiar, less and less of the brain is needed or used or the particular brain region becomes less activated. Think about how much concentration it takes to learn a foreign language and how much easier it becomes over time to speak in that language as the brain becomes more efficient at the task. Dr. Bennett told us, "A good brain is an efficient brain. Cognitive reserve probably has to do with efficiency and the way the brain operates."

A brain with cognitive reserve may have a rich system of "alternative routes" for neural connections. Dr. Bennett compared this to the side streets off a city freeway. "If there is an accident on the freeway, you can get off and use the side streets. You might need to meander around a bit, but you could get where you were going. The side streets weren't built for through traffic, but you can use them for this different purpose. On the other hand, if you're on an isolated two-lane

Working Harder: How the Brain Fights Back

Dr. Randy Buckner, a neuroscientist and psychology professor at Harvard University, studies normal memory during aging. "As we age, our hair thins, our skin wrinkles, and our brain changes

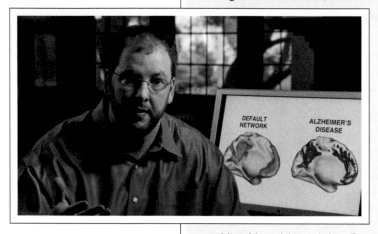

as well. It's not surprising that memory, being one of the highest capacities of the mind, is affected by normal aging." His work explores the brain activity that may underlie the cognitive reserve described by Dr. Bennett in his population studies.

In one area of research, Dr. Buckner is using fMRI images to compare brain function between healthy young people and healthy older adults. Research volunteers memorize a series of words, and then their brains are scanned while they recall the words. "You might expect less brain activity in the older adults, but that's not what we found. There is increased activity across the brain. We think this may be a form of compensation. They are trying to perform as close to normal levels as possible. So they recruit more regions than when they were younger and their brains were more intact."

Dr. Buckner hypothesizes that the ability to draw on the brain's reserves may be one reason some people are able to maintain performance into their eighties and nineties even if there are signs of brain damage or decline.

His idea raises many questions. Why are some people able to call upon these brain reserves to remain cognitively healthy while others experience cognitive decline or dementia? How can science help all individuals make maximum use of the reserve they do have?

highway and there's an accident, you may have no alternate route." Dr. Bennett speculates that a brain with cognitive reserve may have many more pathways and connections, or "alternate routes," that can rewire themselves when challenged by disease. These may prevent a deficit in memory even though there is pathology in the brain.

A more efficient brain may also help a person perform better on cognitive tests. Processing speed, or how quickly one scans and comprehends information, tends to decline with aging. But according to Dr. Bennett, having a conversation, reading a book or newspaper, listening to the radio, and watching TV all involve processing information, and people who spend more time processing greater varieties of information are found to be better able to maintain youthful scores on tests of processing speed. If a person has better processing resources, it might protect her from expressing Alzheimer's pathology as memory loss.

The Role of Education

Cognitive reserve may be linked to a multitude of factors including genetics; early life health, education, and experiences; and other health factors that are still unknown.

Studies have identified factors in early life that correlate with outcomes later in life, including the risk of Alzheimer's disease. This observational research, noted Dr. Richard Hodes, the director of the National Institute on Aging, suggests, for example, "that the number of years of early education, as well as the quality of education, may be protective factors associated with reduced risk of Alzheimer's disease later in life." He called these and other observations "a strong argument for pursuing research, such as clinical trials, to test directly whether specific lifestyle interventions will affect risk for Alzheimer's disease in later years."

Study after study has associated education with protective factors. Scientists often quantify education in years of formal schooling, but it might be more accurate to refer to a cognitively challenging lifetime of work and engagement. This can be present regardless of occupation or level of formal education. Consider how mentally challenging it is to learn to play an instrument or even play a sport.

Crosswords and mind games have received a lot of attention as ways to stay mentally sharp, and even to reduce the risk of AD.

Bennett suggests that the greatest benefit may come from many years of mental stimulation. "How much that will help if you start when you're eighty is not really clear, especially if you were not cognitively active your whole life. The earlier in life you start good cognitive health habits and the more you maintain them, the better off you will probably be over the long run."

Brain Building

Education is the factor that has received by far the most attention among Alzheimer's disease researchers interested in cognitive reserve, because of its strong correlation with cognitive performance noted in the studies described above. However, Dr. Bennett brings a unique perspective to this field of study, and an expansive way of thinking about all the factors that might contribute to the creation of an efficient brain.

One of the out-of-the-box ways that Dr. Bennett has approached thinking about brain activity is to consider how people must develop semantic memory—generalized knowledge that does not involve memory of a specific event—each time they interact with someone they know. Consider that the brain has to work hard to help a person maintain a social network. If a man bumps into an old friend, somebody he hasn't seen in twenty years, he recalls in an instant how he knows her, whether she's married, has children, and so on. This task alone stimulates the brain. Then the old information is integrated with the new information from the current encounter, which is stored in his memory bank so he is able to call it all up again the next time he meets her. People with complex social networks are constantly engaging with others in this way, updating their brain files. Perhaps, like formal education, this stimulates the brain and creates more cognitive reserve.

It turns out that having many friends and participating in social activities have been associated with reduced cognitive decline and decreased risk of dementia in older adults. For example, the National Institute on Aging–funded Memory and Aging Project, which Dr. Bennett directs, found an association between higher levels of social engagement and better cognitive function over time.

Dr. Bennett's other major study, the Religious Orders Study, also has associated a high level of cognitive activity with reduced Alzheimer's disease risk. Investigators on that project periodically asked study participants—older nuns, priests, and religious brothers—to describe how much time they spent in seven information-processing activities: having a conversation, reading a book, listening to the radio, watching television, reading newspapers, playing puzzle games, and going to museums. After following the volunteers for four years, investigators found that the risk of developing AD was, on average, 47 percent lower for participants who did the activities most frequently than for those who did them least frequently. Other studies have shown similar results. In addition, a growing body of research, including other findings from the Religious Orders Study, has associated a higher level of education with increased memory and learning abilities, even when a person has sufficient deposition of beta-amyloid plaques to qualify for a diagnosis of AD.

Because late-life cognitive activity is likely related to lifelong engagement in cognitively stimulating activities, Dr. Bennett and colleagues examined lifelong learning and mentally stimulating activity among participants in the Rush Memory and Aging Project. After following the research volunteers for up to five years, investigators found that both current and past activities were related to risk of AD. Importantly, even after accounting for the effects of past activity, people in the bottom 10 percent for current activity level were nearly three times as likely to develop AD as those in the top 10 percent of activity. Other studies have shown that people who are bilingual or multilingual seem to develop AD at a later age than do people who speak only one language.

Although these findings are provocative, they still need to be interpreted with caution. It's not always possible to tell whether Alzheimer's disease is the cause or the consequence of limited participation in social activities. The disease develops over the course of decades before symptoms appear, and it is possible that early AD could cause a person to limit social or intellectual activities. However, Dr. Bennett did not find a relationship between participation in cognitive activity and AD pathology in the brain. This suggests that the level of cognitive activity was unlikely to be a result of AD and that whatever benefit is derived from cognitive activity is likely the result of its effect on brain reserve.

Personality Factors and Social Networks

In addition to the connection with social networks, brain reserve might also be associated with personality factors. Dr. Bennett's studies have suggested that some personality traits, such as how someone reacts to stress, are associated with cognitive function. "Not how much stress you're under, but how you deal with stress, is associated with the loss of episodic memory, which is a hallmark of Alzheimer's disease." Research suggests, for example, that people who worry a lot or have experienced long-term depression or anxiety have twice the risk of cognitive decline.

Loneliness is another factor. It's not just the size of one's social network that is important, but the ease or difficulty one has making social connections. A pattern of unsatisfying relationships correlates with an increased risk of cognitive decline.

Dr. Bennett speculates that a life of stress, depression, and loneliness changes the brain in ways that we don't yet understand. Perhaps such situations create a negative environment in the brain. "This would not directly cause the pathology of Alzheimer's disease, but it may cause some other type of damage that would make Alzheimer's changes more likely to be expressed as memory loss." Dr. Bennett's research also suggests that an extensive social network—not only how many people one knows, but how many people one knows intimately and feels comfortable confiding in—might be protective in its own way. It could be, Bennett says, that "the larger the network, the less likely people are to decline, the less likely they are to experience clinical Alzheimer's disease."

.   .   .

The connections among education, cognitive stimulation, social engagement, and Alzheimer's disease remain unclear. Additional studies will be needed to determine cause-and-effect relationships—to test, for example, whether mental stimulation as an intervention will directly influence the risk of Alzheimer's disease. Without direct evidence, Dr. Hodes explained, "we are not able to conclude with any certainty that pursuing education, keeping your brain active, or developing an extensive social network specifically will prevent Alzheimer's disease." However, he also noted that a body of research—as well as common sense—shows that many of these activities are good for health and aging and their potential benefits for Alzheimer's disease should be active lines of scientific inquiry.

In this vein, cognitive reserve is an important area of AD research. "We know that proper diet and exercise, weight control, lower salt intake, and eating fresh fruits and vegetables can help reduce the likelihood of cardiovascular disease. Similarly, we are trying to determine what people can do in their lives to maintain cognitive health within their genetic constraints," Dr. Bennett told us. "What can we do as young people, as middle-aged people, and even as older people to create brains that would tolerate AD pathology if it developed? As you take your brain into your ninth and tenth decade, it's likely to be assaulted by a variety of insults such as Alzheimer's changes and strokes. You want the most robust, efficient, rapid-decision-making, multi-tasking brain you possibly can have, because that may allow you to maintain your cognition, despite all the other things that could happen to it."

TWO COMMUNITY-BASED INVESTIGATIONS

The **Religious Orders Study** is a community-based investigation of more than eleven hundred nuns, priests, and brothers from across the United States who have agreed to be tested every year. It has been funded by the National Institute on Aging since 1993. Participants do not have dementia when they enter the study, and they agree to be organ donors at the time of death.

Dr. Bennett studies religious communities because of their relative homogeneity. "In a sense, we have a captive audience: this is a large group of people living communally with fairly similar lifestyles." Many participants are old. Many die before they develop memory loss. Some develop MCI, some develop Alzheimer's disease, and some never develop cognitive impairments. The study allows Dr. Bennett to see people age and develop Alzheimer's disease in the context of their lives. "We want to understand the disease and all the factors leading up to it, in terms of how these individuals lived."

A comprehensive assessment of the participant's current living situation is made, as is a careful survey of her life history. Interviewers capture information about the

Examining brain tissue taken on autopsy from a participant in the Religious Orders Study.

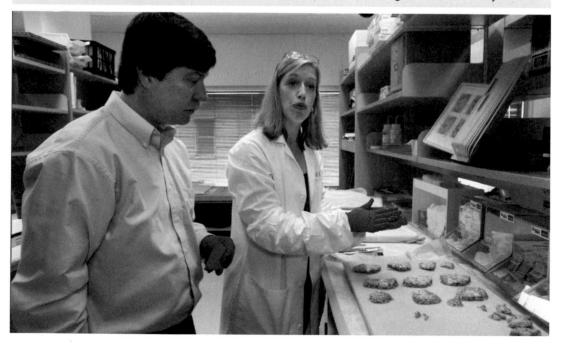

occupation, education, and socioeconomic status of each person's parents. They also ask questions about how the person grew up: birth order, how many books and newspapers were in the house, or whether the family visited the library. Using archives and census data, they check literacy rates and socioeconomic status among the people who were living in the same neighborhoods as the volunteers at various stages of their life: childhood, young adulthood, and middle age. They also collect information on life challenges and trauma to assess levels of psychological stress. Among many other illuminating results, data from the Religious Orders Study have shown that engaging in mentally stimulating activity is correlated with delaying the onset of AD and slowing the rate at which people lose cognitive function.

Sister Alice Caulfield, of the Sisters of Charity of the Blessed Virgin Mary in Dubuque, Iowa, is participating in the study because she wants to help science. "Since we've started the study, I do believe they've learned many new things about Alzheimer's disease. They certainly don't have a cure, but they're beginning to figure out factors that might indicate how this disease takes place. The scientists are educating other people, using our brains to help that. Whatever they can learn from us is of value to the world."

Dr. Bennett also directs the **Rush Memory and Aging Project,** a community-based

Sister Alice Caulfield

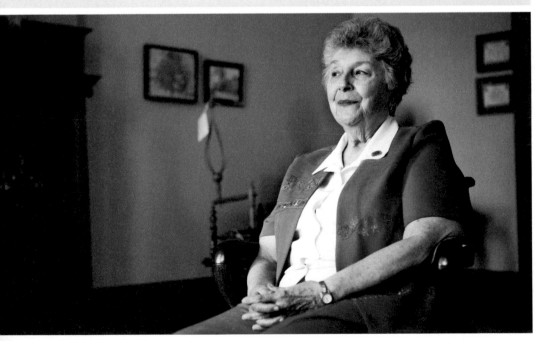

investigation of more than twelve hundred older people from across northeastern Illinois. It is funded by the National Institute on Aging and has been ongoing since 1997. Participants do not have dementia when they enter the study, agree to be tested every year, and consent to donate their brains, spinal cords, and selected muscles and nerves at the time of death.

In contrast to studies in religious communities, participants in the Rush Memory and Aging Project are much more representative of the older population in general in terms of background, education, and life experiences. "We are interested in how life experiences affect cognitive and motor function in late life and how they affect changes in the brain and other parts of the nervous system," Dr. Bennett said. The study allows his team to see people age mentally and physically in the context in which they live. "We want to understand all the factors involved in the full spectrum of problems associated with aging."

Dr. Bennett is interested in characterizing the cognitive milieu within which a person was born, grew up, and grew old. Thus, the interviewers capture information about each person's parents and the community in which they were born. Researchers determine the participants' current level of physical activity by having them wear a device the size of a wristwatch that measures how much each participant moves over the course of ten days. They also collect data on eating habits.

In addition to studying the effects of early life experiences, diet, and exercise, Dr. Bennett is interested in determining how cognitive abilities affect real-world decision-making. With this goal in mind, the study also captures information on the ability of participants to make informed choices about health and financial matters, as well as details on their decision-making styles. Among many other illuminating results, data from the Rush Memory and Aging Project have shown that people with larger social networks are less likely to manifest memory loss despite the accumulation of Alzheimer's disease pathology. Another surprising finding made by Dr. Bennett and his colleagues suggests that many factors associated with the risk of AD are also associated with loss of mobility, which implies that loss of cognitive and motor abilities may share common causes and that slowing down cognitive decline may also improve physical health.

11

ASSESSING THE POTENTIAL BENEFITS OF EXERCISE AND DIET

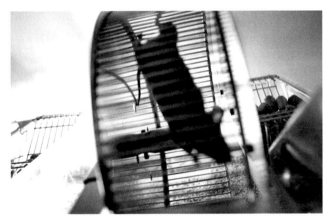

Regular exercise and a healthy diet reduce the risk of vascular disease and diabetes because they help keep blood pressure, blood glucose, blood cholesterol, and weight at normal levels. Since these diseases and their underlying conditions have associations with Alzheimer's disease, could exercise and diet also help reduce the risk of Alzheimer's disease and improve brain health and function in general?

Dr. Richard Hodes of the NIA summarized the overall state of research into exercise and cognitive function: "There is enormous interest now in what effects lifestyle interventions, such as exercise and diet, may have on the risk for Alzheimer's disease, or on brain health and function in general. There is, in fact, a good deal of evidence bearing on this. Some of it comes from observations in epidemiological studies. For example, adults who are physically active appear to be at decreased risk of Alzheimer's disease. The association is suggestive, although it doesn't provide, as yet, a definitive link.

"At the same time, there is recent evidence in animal models suggesting that exercise and diet can modify the progression of Alzheimer's disease pathology, evidence that there may be a mechanism by which interventions can actually prevent the advance of lesions, which are a model for the pathology of Alzheimer's disease. We have observations in humans suggesting that similar lifestyle variables are associated with greater or reduced risk of Alzheimer's disease. This convergence provides a real possibility that lifestyle changes in people will have a positive outcome on their risk of Alzheimer's disease. We are now at the stage of taking this convergence of suggestive evidence to more definitive clinical trials."

With the greater strength and specificity of evidence that might come from clinical trials, Dr. Hodes explained, we should be able to determine whether and what types of exercise and diet are beneficial, and at what point in life they might make the most difference. While these studies are under way, we should engage in lifestyle interventions demonstrated to be safe and effective for healthy aging and to reduce the risk of other age-related conditions. Dr. Hodes encourages exercise and a healthy diet, for example, for both their known and potential benefits.

Exercise and the Brain

Recent large-scale observational studies in various groups, including nurses, people living in rural areas, and older adults, have found reduced risk of cognitive decline and dementia among those who exercised regularly. These findings provide much valuable information but can't tell us whether a cause-and-effect relationship exists between exercise and Alzheimer's disease risk. Other factors may be involved; for example, people who exercise may also have a more healthful diet or take better care of their health in other ways. Epidemiological studies like these need to be followed by other kinds of research, such as controlled clinical trials, to reinforce the findings and explore the reasons behind them.

Dr. Carl Cotman, a biochemist and the director of both the Institute for Brain Aging and Dementia at the University of California Irvine and the Alzheimer's Disease Center there, has focused much of his long career on how the brain ages and how lifestyle interventions might influence that process. He is fascinated by how the brain withstands the pressures of the aging process.

"The fact that a neuron has to live for a lifetime is a real challenge to a cell," Dr. Cotman said. "Most cells in the body don't have an infinite lifetime. The one-hundred-year-old neuron is a hero to me because it's self-repairing. It doesn't get to jump out of the circuit and get fixed at the local doctor or the local garage. It has to be maintained, and it does this through self-repair mechanisms. It's looking out for its own future while it maintains its own performance. That's a real triumph."

One of the mechanisms by which neurons repair themselves involves BDNF, or brain-derived neurotrophic factor, a protein that supports the survival of existing neurons and encourages the development of new ones. Dr. Cotman wondered if BDNF might help

Dr. Carl Cotman

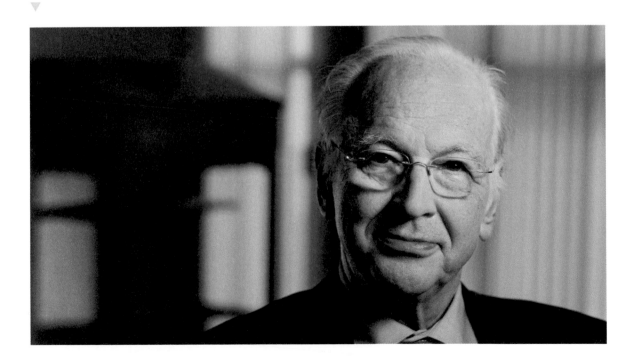

increase the longevity of neurons and prevent cognitive decline. "What would be the most ideal change that you could induce in the brain to help it maintain function longer and learn better? Several years ago, I thought it might be exercise. At the time, we knew that exercise improved muscle function, but there wasn't literature to show that it would have any impact on the brain beyond causing it to burn more energy. However, I thought that a growth factor like BDNF, a kind of a nutrient or a fertilizer to neurons, might be naturally increased with exercise."

He and his colleagues conducted a series of studies on rats to test that hypothesis. They separated them into two groups: an active group in cages with exercise wheels and a sedentary group in cages without exercise wheels. When his team examined the brains of the physically active animals, they found that levels of BDNF had increased not so much in the regions related to motor and sensory functions, which might have been expected, but, surprisingly, in the regions most integral to thinking and learning. These same regions are vulnerable to aging and AD. "The brain knew how to look out for itself in a way we had had no idea about. It has a self-preservation mechanism that allows it to learn better."

Another study looked for behavioral changes. "We know that a mouse bred to develop AD finds it more and more difficult to learn as it ages. We wanted to know whether exercise improved the ability to learn." The mice were provided with exercise wheels when they were young. In late middle age, their learning and memory were challenged with a water maze. "It tests their ability to identify a particular space in a big area." At first, through trial and error, mice find an "invisible" platform located just below the surface in a pool of water made opaque by adding powdered milk. In subsequent trials, the mice use geometric shapes and symbols situated around the maze to recall how to navigate to the platform. "It's very similar to what you do when you're trying to find your car in a parking lot. You can't see your car, so you have to use cues around you to identify the correct location. The mice utilize the cues around the maze to find the platform. When they stand on it, they're happy because they're not wet anymore and they're not cold." The mice that had exercised were quickly able to remember the platform's location on later attempts, whereas the sedentary animals swam in circles, unable to locate the platform.

For a follow-up study, transgenic mice (specially bred to express

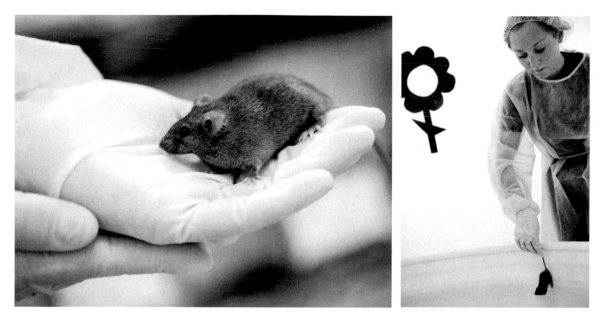

▲

LEFT: *One of the transgenic mice Dr. Cotman uses to study exercise and the role of BDNF in learning and memory.*

RIGHT: *The water maze tests the ability of the mouse to remember the location of a hidden platform; the mouse can use images like the flower as navigational clues.*

a mutant gene associated with the development of AD) began exercising late in life, when they had already developed AD pathology. "Much to our surprise and delight, the exercise effect worked even after the animals had a fair amount of pathology." Dr. Cotman found less accumulation of beta-amyloid in the brains of the mice that had been allowed to exercise throughout their lives, and even in those that began to run later in life, compared to the amount of beta-amyloid in sedentary animals.

Dr. Cotman's follow-up studies have suggested that an increased level of BDNF may improve the ability of nerve cells to receive signals. He has discovered that BDNF builds synaptic structures, and he and others have shown that BDNF induces the growth of bud-like structures called spines on the dendrites that extend out from the nerve cell body. An increased number of spines allow neurons to signal to each other more efficiently.

In older rats and mice, other research has found that exercise increases the number of small vessels that supply blood to the brain. The brain benefits by having more energy for its metabolic functions from greater vascular flow.

Animal studies help explain the associations identified in epidemiological studies, but there is no guarantee that the same interventions will work with people. The National Institute on Aging has

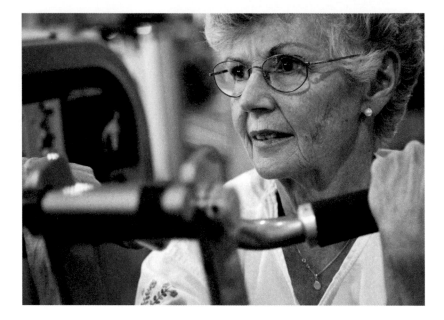

supported several clinical studies to define the biological basis of the possible effects of exercise. To assess brain changes, one trial used fMRI imaging to measure changes in brain activity in older adults before and after a six-month program of brisk walking. Results showed that brain activity increased in specific brain regions as cardiovascular fitness increased. A similar trial showed that brain volume increased as a result of a walking program. These findings support the observational studies and suggest a biological basis for the role of aerobic exercise in helping maintain cognitive function in aging adults, at least in the short term. Other clinical trials are investigating the effects of exercise in cognitively healthy older people, people at risk of MCI, and people with MCI.

Diet and the Brain

A diet rich in fruits, vegetables, and whole grains, and low in fats and added sugars, can reduce the risk of heart disease, diabetes, and obesity. Can certain dietary patterns or components also help preserve cognitive function and reduce the risk of Alzheimer's disease?

Epidemiological studies have suggested that consuming foods rich in antioxidants—such as brightly colored fruits and dark green,

Exercise and the Dentate Gyrus

Dr. Scott Small, an energetic neurologist at Columbia University, is trying to pinpoint exactly where in the brain exercise has the most beneficial impact. In Chapter 5, we learned about his studies of early changes in the hippocampal formation in Alzheimer's disease, but his research on exercise is also intriguing.

He and his team conducted a study that allowed mice to run freely in exercise cages. Researchers monitored their activity level so it could later be correlated with the test results. Using fMRI imaging, Dr. Small found that within the hippocampal formation, the dentate gyrus seemed to benefit most from exercise. This is the region of the brain that loses function in age-related memory loss.

Since the molecules that make up the dentate gyrus are thought to be similar in mice and humans, Dr. Small thought that exercise might have a similar beneficial effect in humans. "We've recently used imaging techniques to find that physical exercise has a selective effect in the dentate gyrus in humans.

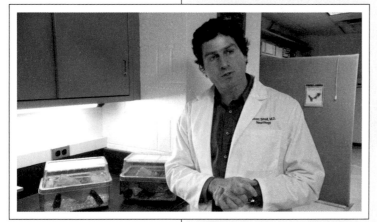

This immediately suggests that perhaps physical exercise might be a good way to ameliorate normal age-related changes. Based on that, we're now designing a study to see if physical exercise really reduces the memory loss that occurs with aging by selectively improving function in the dentate gyrus."

Although BDNF might be playing a role, Dr. Small does not know what is mediating the exercise effect that he observes. "We hope to identify the key proteins that respond to exercise. The next step would be to develop compounds that can ameliorate age-related memory decline." This possible drug target would be especially helpful to people who cannot engage in aerobic exercise and create molecular changes on their own.

Dr. Scott Small with some of the mice in his exercise study.

leafy vegetables—may be one way to preserve cognition. Antioxidants, molecules capable of slowing the oxidation of other molecules, are thought to reduce cell damage throughout the body by counteracting free radicals, highly reactive molecules that are by-products of energy production in all cells. With age, either more free radicals are produced, or they are not cleared away as efficiently. They can accumulate in neurons in the brain, causing loss of function. Dr. Cotman describes this oxidative damage as "something like molecular rust." Free radicals occur throughout the body, but the brain's high metabolic rate and long-lived neurons make it particularly vulnerable. The destructive nature of free radicals in the aging brain is yet another focus of AD research.

A team at Harvard Medical School explored the possible benefits of foods high in antioxidants by analyzing epidemiological data from more than thirteen thousand participants aged seventy and older in the Nurses' Health Study. They found that the women who reported eating the greatest amounts of green leafy vegetables (spinach, kale, and romaine lettuce) and cruciferous vegetables (broccoli, cabbage, brussel sprouts, and cauliflower) experienced a slower rate of cognitive decline than women who said they ate the smallest amounts of these vegetables. The apparent benefits of antioxidants remained high even when the scientists accounted for other factors that might have influenced the results, such as the use of vitamins, physical activity, smoking, alcohol consumption, and educational level. Eating fruit did not appear to be associated with improved cognitive ability. The researchers speculated that the high levels of antioxidants and folate (a nutrient that also appears to be important for proper neural activity and cognitive function) in the green leafy and cruciferous vegetables were responsible.

Other epidemiological studies have looked at the whole diet rather than particular components. Studies of adults in Manhattan, for example, link the "Mediterranean diet"—which includes lots of fruits, vegetables, and bread; low to moderate amounts of dairy, fish, poultry, and red wine; small amounts of red meat; and frequent use of olive oil—with a reduced risk of AD and longer survival of people who already had the disease.

Researchers have turned to animal studies to explore the link between diet and AD more directly. In one study conducted on transgenic mice, scientists have found that curcumin, an ingredient in curry that has strong antioxidant and anti-inflammatory properties, prevented the aggregation of beta-amyloid peptides into oligomers and inhibited the toxic effect of these oligomers. Other teams have found that a diet high in DHA, an omega-3 fatty acid found in fish, also reduced beta-amyloid and plaque levels in the brains of transgenic mice. These results are now being tested in a number of clinical trials that are examining the effects of specific dietary components on cognitive decline and AD.

Dr. Cotman and his collaborators have demonstrated that old dogs are for many reasons an even more useful model for this type of research than transgenic mice. Dogs experience cognitive decline as they age and can be tested with cognitive challenges similar to those used in higher-order primates and humans. More importantly, their brains naturally accumulate beta-amyloid plaques that are identical to those in people, and the amount of beta-amyloid deposits correlates with the severity of their cognitive decline.

Dr. Cotman collaborated with a research team at the University of Toronto, headed by Dr. William Milgram, to conduct several studies with aged beagles to determine whether an antioxidant-rich diet would improve the dogs' cognitive function, learning ability, and memory. The research team fed the beagles exactly the same diet for three years. ("Try that in a human," Dr. Cotman said. "Nobody is going to eat the same thing for breakfast, lunch, and dinner for three years, but the dogs were fine with it.") The diet was enriched with antioxidants, vitamins E and C, and fruit and vegetable extracts.

The beagles were divided into four groups. A first group was put on the antioxidant supplement diet. The second group had an enriched environment with novel toys and a cage companion, as well as additional opportunities to exercise, but no dietary changes. The third group had both the antioxidant-enriched diet and the enriched environment. The fourth group was a control, provided with a regular diet and a standard environment.

Over the three years, the dogs were given a series of behavioral tests similar to cognitive tests used in research with humans and primates. Even in the first few months of the study, the team saw short-term improvements on some of the learning tests. "We were shocked," Dr. Cotman told us.

"When we began the study, the beagles were between eight and eleven years of age—late-middle age for a dog. We picked this age because we wanted to see if we could make a difference as they aged. At year one, we gave them a hard learning task. None of the animals

Diet, Insulin Resistance, and Cognition

We learned about Dr. Suzanne Craft's research into the association between diabetes and Alzheimer's disease in Chapter 8. As part of that research, she is studying the impact of diet.

A diet high in saturated fat and sugar increases the risk of developing insulin resistance because blood glucose causes a rise in insulin, and "a high-fat diet raises insulin levels and increases the number of fat cells, both of which work together to reduce the body's ability to respond to insulin."

To study the earliest changes through which insulin resistance might increase the risk of Alzheimer's disease, Dr. Craft and her team developed a way to cause temporary insulin resistance in order to study its effects. One group of participants consumed a high-fat/high-sugar diet for four weeks, while a second group ate a low-fat/low-sugar diet. The high-fat diet used in this experiment is a diet that many Americans consume (a typical "bad" Western diet), with 45 percent of calories coming from fat (most from saturated fat) and a high sugar content. The researchers did not add to the amount of calories a person would normally consume; they just increased the proportion of those calories that came from saturated fat and sugar. Not surprisingly, this group experienced substantial increases in LDL cholesterol, the type that clogs arteries. The degree of change was striking considering that they had followed the diet for only a month. In addition, tests of their spinal fluid showed changes in beta-amyloid levels and markers for inflammation, both of which are associated with AD.

The participants who followed the low-fat diet ate foods low in saturated fats, and all the fats were healthy fats, like olive oil. The diet was also low in simple sugars, with complex carbohydrates coming from fruits, vegetables, and whole grains. Compared to the high-fat/high-sugar diet group, this group had lower insulin levels, lower levels of LDL cholesterol, and improved beta-amyloid and inflammation profiles in their spinal fluid. "Even four weeks of eating well produced a benefit for these individuals in terms of their insulin resistance and their beta-amyloid profile."

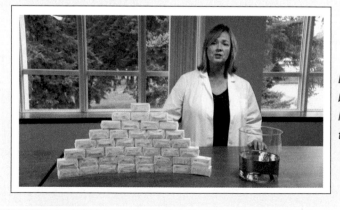

Dr. Craft comparing the amount of butter used in one month of the MEAL study's high-fat "Western" diet to the olive oil used in the low-fat diet.

could perform it. At year two, we started to see an improvement in the animals that were in the combined enrichment and diet group. By year three, the animals on the combined enrichment and antioxidant diet were able to perform the task, but the others still couldn't do it." (The animals that received the enriched diet alone and the behavior enrichment alone also showed improvement—just not as much as those in the group that received both.)

Dr. Cotman took this to mean that this group had gained function. "They were now performing almost as well as a group of younger animals." The study received a good deal of press coverage, and one publication described the results as: "You can teach an old dog new tricks." Dr. Cotman agreed that "it's what we did. We taught an old dog new tricks."

"I'd like to believe that you could teach an old individual new tricks, as well. I'm trying to practice this myself. For instance, I'm learning how to play tennis, which I didn't really know how to do a couple of years ago. So I'm learning a new trick, so to speak—and I'm doing okay at it."

12

DEVELOPING NEW DRUG TREATMENTS

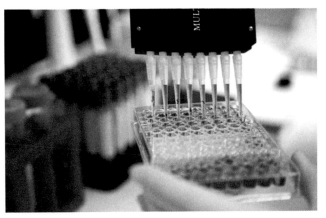

The most crucial prerequisite for successful drug development to treat any disease is to have identified specific targets against which therapies can be directed. In the last two decades, scientists have identified a number of therapeutic targets specific to Alzheimer's disease. The discovery of the three genes that invariably cause early-onset AD and of ApoE-ε4, the first and most significant susceptibility gene for late-onset AD, have lent a great deal of strength to the beta-amyloid hypothesis. The importance of these genetic findings resides in the fact that these four genes all act on the same cascade of events: through various mechanisms, they all lead to an increase in the buildup of beta-amyloid and neurofibrillary tangles in the brain, which eventually causes neurons to die. This convergence of evidence pointed toward beta-amyloid as a major therapeutic target.

Hundreds of laboratories around the world are contributing knowledge about the role of beta-amyloid in AD. Each in a multitude of increasingly understood steps in the beta-amyloid cascade might become a site to target with promising therapeutic compounds.

Dr. Paul Aisen, director of the Alzheimer's Disease Cooperative Study—a long-standing, National Institute on Aging–backed initiative to coordinate clinical trials of promising drugs that may be outside the purview of pharmaceutical companies—described the encouraging tenor of this era in AD drug development: "Everybody's coming together now. It's a huge endeavor, but we're working together to make progress, so that now we have candidate drugs that target the specific process that's initiating Alzheimer's disease, we have brought them into human trials, and we are perhaps close to success."

Like many others in the field, Dr. Aisen believes that researchers are well on track toward reaching their goals. "We need to optimize

Dr. Paul Aisen

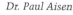

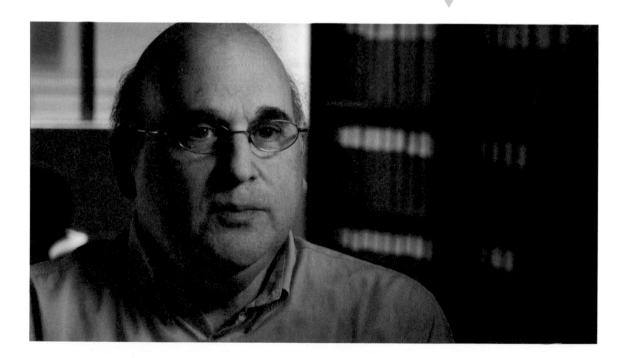

the treatment of the symptoms, but even more importantly, we need to slow the disease process. We need to halt it. We need to be able to prevent the development of Alzheimer's disease. We need to promote healthy aging—aging without memory impairment, without Alzheimer's disease."

These are undoubtedly ambitious objectives. Many drug targets are being investigated. Clinical trials of ninety-one drugs were under way as of 2008. More drug candidates are awaiting Food and Drug Administration approval to enter human testing. Promising drugs may help people with AD maintain their mental functioning. Others may slow, delay, or even prevent AD. Inside the world of AD drug research today, the optimism is palpable, but scientists also realize that significant challenges remain to be overcome.

The First Drugs

In the mid-1970s, scientists discovered that the levels of the neurotransmitter acetylcholine, which neurons in the hippocampal formation and cerebral cortex use when they form memories, were sharply lower in people with Alzheimer's disease. This was one of the first discoveries that linked AD to a biochemical change in the brain.

In 1985, there was a small trial of a medication that would stop the breakdown of acetylcholine. This launched further trials, which had the support of the National Institutes of Health, the Alzheimer's Association, the academic world, and the pharmaceutical industry. This drug, tacrine (Cognex®), was approved by the FDA for clinical use in 1993; it modestly improved memory in people with AD, but had significant side effects on liver function. Tacrine has since been superseded by four other drugs, three of which operate on the same principle of maintaining acetylcholine levels—donepezil (Aricept®), rivastigmine (Exelon®), galantamine (Razadyne®)—and a fourth, memantine (Namenda®), which targets another brain chemical known as glutamate. These drugs have been approved to treat symptoms of mild, moderate, and severe AD. These medications help some people maintain cognitive abilities, and they can help address some behavioral symptoms as well. However, they appear to be effective for only a few months to perhaps a few years, and none affects the progressive, degenerative AD process.

The Stages of Drug Development

The development of drugs for Alzheimer's disease, like all drug development, must move through research and regulatory stages that typically take ten to twelve years. A single drug trial in AD involves hundreds of professionals and can cost hundreds of millions of dollars.

Before a new drug comes to market and can be prescribed by physicians, it passes through multiple steps of testing and optimization for both efficacy and safety in animal models, followed by clinical trials with people. The process begins when a researcher identifies a potential drug target, for example, a protein or a process that may be involved in a disease. Lab experiments in test tubes, tissue cultures, and animal models must demonstrate why a target should be investigated. **Dr. William Thies,** the chief medical and scientific officer of the Alzheimer's Association, said, "A scientist discovers a chemical or biological reaction involved in the pathology of Alzheimer's disease and that opens up the possibility that we can interfere with this reaction or alter the molecule to produce a desirable outcome giving hope that we can generate a therapy."

Not every compound works out, as most of them do not have desirable drug-like properties. They may be highly toxic, insoluble, impure, or unstable. "They may not be able to travel into the part of the body that needs them; in this case, they must cross the blood-brain barrier. Also, ideally drug administration should be easy."

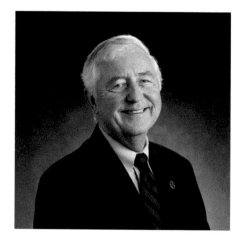

Dr. William Thies

When a pathway has been discovered and there is evidence that a promising chemical can alter it to produce a desirable effect, medicinal chemists work to design a compound that will have the necessary properties of a drug. Biologists and physiologists then test the safety and efficacy of the substance in cells, tissue cultures, and animals. If the investigators believe that the drug is safe enough for humans and might potentially be effective, they apply to the FDA for an Investigational New Drug (IND) designation for permission to begin human testing. If approved, the compound moves to the last step of development—clinical studies in humans, which compare the experimental treatment to a placebo (an inactive pill) or to a standard treatment.

Clinical trials have three stages, which are determined by the drug approval process outlined by the FDA. During Phase I, the research team administers the treatment to a small number of people and carefully observes how it acts in the body and whether it is safe. Typically, healthy volunteers participate in Phase I trials, but sometimes people with the disease are involved. The purpose of this phase is to establish the highest dose people can tolerate before experiencing harmful side effects. In Alzheimer's disease studies, Phase I usually lasts a few months until a range of safe doses is determined. When that is accomplished, researchers may decide to pursue Phase II testing in actual patients.

More people are involved in a Phase II trial, and they take the treatment for a longer time. The goals of Phase II are to test safety still further. Dr. Thies told us, "You also begin to look for evidence of effectiveness. Typically, that evidence is not statistically significant, but you want to see if you can detect a signal that the drug effect is present. If you're giving an inadequate dose you won't get any effect. And if you're giving too big a dose, you will probably aggravate side effects."

A Phase III trial is a much larger study that establishes that the drug is safe and has the power to produce the desired effect. If successful, the trial may be replicated to confirm the findings. If the results from Phase III demonstrate safety and statistically significant efficacy, researchers may submit their data to the FDA for approval of the drug. The FDA provides consultation at all levels of human testing, and experts there review the results of Phase III and decide whether to allow the treatment to be marketed for prescription use. In the case of a potentially disease-modifying drug for AD, regulators there would likely designate the application for priority review, since the drug would address unmet medical needs. Such a priority designation sets the target date for FDA action on the application at six months, as opposed to the year or longer that is a more typical timeframe.

As of April 2009, no disease-modifying drugs for AD have received FDA approval. Of the ninety-one drugs currently in clinical trials, more than a dozen are in Phase III.

Drugs in Development

The first step in drug development is actually the most important—picking the right target. "Plaques being deposited, synaptic function being disrupted, mitochondria being damaged, and transport mechanisms changing. It is a challenge to pick the right target," Dr. Aisen explained.

Much drug research is focused on beta-amyloid. Drugs are being developed to prevent its buildup into plaques through slowing or stopping beta-amyloid production, enhancing its removal, inhibiting the clumping of beta-amyloid into oligomers and plaques, and dissolving existing plaques altogether. A number of other ongoing clinical trials are testing specific agents that target the two enzymes that cleave the amyloid precursor protein (APP) into shorter fragments, one of which is beta-amyloid. The beta-amyloid cascade hypothesis suggests that those enzymes, when they cut APP to form beta-amyloid, execute the inciting event in a chain that may ultimately lead to AD.

Two of those enzymes, beta-secretase and gamma-secretase, are believed to work together to create the beta-amyloid peptides that form plaques in the brain, and are two of the points of intervention targeted by current drug development efforts. Until recently, beta-secretase had been difficult to work with because its shape does not lend itself easily to drug development. Finally, in early 2008, the results of the initial human testing of a drug candidate to inhibit beta-secretase showed that the treatment was safe and well tolerated by healthy volunteers and led to a reduction in beta-amyloid levels in the plasma. Unlike beta-secretase, gamma-secretase is not a single molecule, but a complex of molecules. Because of this, it may be easier to interfere with its function since its complexity provides many potential targets. But gamma-secretase is essential to many other biological processes in the body, and any potential drug targeting its role in beta-amyloid production would have to work in a way that allows the enzyme to continue to perform its other normal functions.

Additional drug development efforts focus on the beta-amyloid peptide itself. One of the beta-amyloid-busting therapies farthest along in the drug development process is a vaccine currently being tested by Elan Pharmaceuticals, an innovative approach that we'll describe in depth later in the chapter.

Other broad strategies researchers are pursuing include attempts to prevent brain cell dysfunction and death by slowing oxidative stress, averting inflammation, or maintaining blood flow; increasing levels of neuroprotective molecules in the brain; or preserving the intricate network of connections among neurons. Dr. Lennart Mucke, a scientist recognized in the field for approaching Alzheimer's disease from as many angles as possible, thinks that, "in the future we will treat it like we treat other multi-factorial diseases. We will treat it like we treat hypertension, where, as a physician, you try to get away with giving the patient one drug that they can tolerate. Often you can't control the hypertension with one drug, because you get side effects, so you add another drug that has a mechanistically different route of attack. I believe that in the end, since Alzheimer's disease is so multifactorial, we will probably treat it with combinations of drugs. And I wouldn't be surprised if different patients required different combinations."

This suggests that the right path for Alzheimer's disease drug development is to follow every possible avenue and not just the ones that seem most likely to work. As Dr. Marcelle Morrison-Bogorad, the director of the Division of Neuroscience at the National Institute on Aging, made clear, "Even if the beta-amyloid hypothesis is correct, it doesn't mean that beta-amyloid is going to be the best or the only point of intervention for drug development. It could be tau, or a number of other therapeutic targets. The results of early-stage clinical trials targeting tau look promising and will be further tested in larger clinical trials."

As the largest funder of research into AD, the National Institute on Aging takes this multifactorial view of the disease very seriously. Dr. Morrison-Bogorad added, "Each piece of the puzzle is a possible intervention target. So our policy at the NIA is to cast a broad net and fund many promising avenues of research apart from beta-amyloid aimed at uncovering processes that contribute to the transition between normal aging and pathological changes resulting in Alzheimer's dementia. In parallel, in the past five years, we have developed a robust translational research program that supports the discovery and development of new treatments for AD aimed at multiple therapeutic targets to the stage when they can be tested in human trials supported either by the government or the private sector."

Dr. Aisen sees more collaboration among the many organizations and individuals that participate in the drug development process than ever before. Academic scientists at medical schools are working together with industry scientists at pharmaceutical companies, regulators at the FDA and international regulatory agencies, funding sources such as the National Institutes of Health, and advocates such as the Alzheimer's Association to speed up the pace of research and encourage the exploration of new ideas, drug compounds, and biomarkers.

The Alzheimer's Disease Cooperative Study of the National

Institute on Aging is a consortium of clinical trial centers across the country. The federal government funds many trials, especially those that might not be of great interest to large pharmaceutical companies because of patent issues that minimize their profit potential. The study selects new compounds for human testing that were developed

Volunteers Needed

A typical Phase III clinical trial may include anywhere from a few hundred to several thousand participants. Usually it takes one to two years to find enough volunteers for such a large study. Ultimately, the success of Alzheimer's disease drug development depends on having enough volunteers for each of the clinical trial phases. "No matter how rapidly science moves forward," Dr. Aisen observed, "no matter how many terrific molecules are created, no matter how much understanding we have of the disease and how to control it, we will not get a drug to market without large-scale clinical trials that prove it works and it's safe. Without the cooperation of individuals and their families, we will not progress to treatments. There is no way to skip that step. We need many, many people to volunteer their time generously."

People with AD, MCI, or a family history of AD, as well as healthy people with no memory problems or family history of AD, are needed for these trials. In surveys, volunteers generally say that the experience has been positive and express satisfaction at being part of the process that will develop better treatments. The sites conducting the trials have compassionate, skilled, and knowledgeable staff; volunteers get the best standard of care, and often develop a strong relationship with the experts conducting the study. Volunteers also learn about the disease and advances in the field.

Even with all its benefits, volunteering for a clinical trial is a big commitment. After careful review of the possible risks and benefits, volunteers sign an informed consent and are screened to determine if they qualify to participate. During a Phase III AD drug trial, participants may take a pill for eighteen months or longer without knowing whether it is the active treatment or a placebo. An experimental drug may or may not have a benefit and may carry some risk. Participants also agree to have brain scans, blood tests, and in some cases spinal taps, which can require multiple visits to the research center.

"These are brave individuals," Dr. Aisen said, "who participate because they understand there is no other way to move drug development forward. They want to help their children and later generations."

The National Institute on Aging leads the federal government's AD clinical trials effort. To find out more about them, talk to your health care provider, contact the National Institute on Aging's ADEAR Center at 1-800-438-4380, or visit: www.nia.nih.gov/Alzheimers/ResearchInformation/ClinicalTrials.

by individual investigators or small companies that don't have the resources for clinical development, as well as existing medications (such as statins) that are currently used to treat other diseases but that may be useful for the treatment of AD. The study also tests the usefulness of promising nutritional supplements.

"We are currently studying DHA, an omega-3 fatty acid found in fish," Dr. Aisen told us. "Similarly, we have studied antioxidants and herbal extracts. We find that some have a benefit, some don't, and some have unexpected risk. Until you do the rigorously designed controlled clinical trials, you don't know what's going to help and what's going to hurt."

Searching for a Vaccine

One of the more unusual and encouraging approaches scientists are investigating involves a vaccine and antibodies against beta-amyloid plaques. Immunizing people against diseases, such as the measles or influenza, is a common medical practice used to prevent diseases caused by bacteria or viruses. In active immunization, a weakened form of a bacterium or virus is injected into a person, whose immune system then responds by making antibodies to that foreign body. At a later time, if any live bacteria or virus should enter the body, the antibodies present as the result of the immunization find it, bind to it, and draw scavenger cells to attack and destroy it.

In an attempt to rid the brain of beta-amyloid plaques, **Dr. Dale Schenk** hypothesized that it might be possible to vaccinate people against beta-amyloid and use the body's own immune system to treat or prevent AD. Dr. Schenk and his team at Elan Pharmaceuticals were the first research group to explore this possibility.

When the first transgenic mouse model of AD was developed, scientists at Elan came up with a list of experiments they wanted to run in the animals. Since only a small supply of these mice existed at that time, the team ranked the ideas according to their likelihood of success. Dr. Schenk's notion that they test a possible vaccine on the mice was deemed so unlikely to succeed that the team ranked it last. But, as Dr. Dora Games, a member of that research team, described, "The idea was just intriguing enough that eventually we were able to eke out enough mice to perform the experiment."

Dr. Schenk told us that when they did finally carry out the vaccine test, "We found that if mice were vaccinated with beta-amyloid, their immune systems made antibodies against it." As Dr. Schenk predicted, these antibodies attracted the specialized cells called microglia to the plaques, in an effort to clear beta-amyloid debris from the brain. "These scavenger cells saw the plaque as a foreign invader. They were given a signal to get rid of it and they did." The results were so startling that Dr. Schenk thought they were too good to be true. Over several years, he and his team repeated the experiment with a large number of older mice that had developed more plaques. They again found that the amount of plaque decreased in the treated mice, and that other plaque-associated damage, such as inflammation and abnormal cell processes, declined after the immunization.

This opened up the possibility of a human vaccine. Elan Pharmaceuticals and Wyeth collaborated to create the first beta-amyloid vaccine, and a number of other scientific groups confirmed their startling results. Following additional studies in animals, the scientists began small clinical trials to test the safety and efficacy of this vaccine in humans. However, the Phase II trial had to be halted early because a small subset (6 percent) of the 372 participants developed life-threatening brain inflammation in response to the treatment. After the study was cut short, the researchers discovered that 59 of

Dr. Dale Schenk

▼

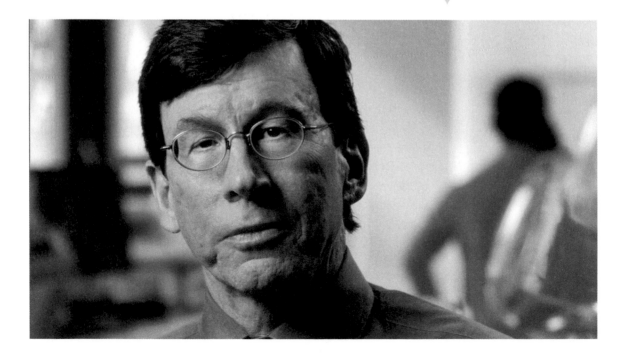

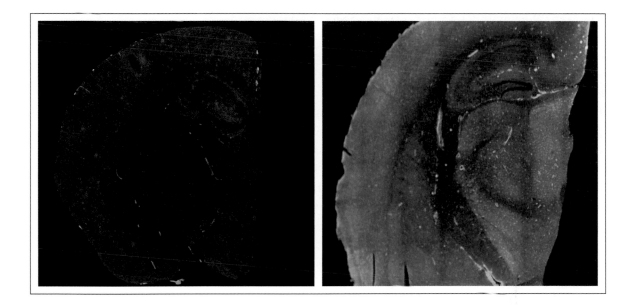

The red signal in the first image shows the presence of beta-amyloid in a brain slice from a mouse model of AD that has not been administered an anti-beta-amyloid antibody. The second image shows the brain of an age-matched mouse six months after treatment with an antibody (passive immunotherapy).

the 372 participants had mounted an immune response to the vaccine injections they received. The research team followed these 59 people for four and a half years after the trial. In a dramatic turn, those participants who had displayed an immune response after being immunized—and who subsequently died of unrelated causes—performed better on some tests of cognitive function and were shown upon autopsy to have had reduced plaque levels in their brain tissue. These results convinced Dr. Schenk to judge the original vaccine trial as a proof of concept. "What we saw in our animal model turned out to be true in people, which means that immunotherapy has the potential to reduce pathology that is already there."

The reports of Dr. Schenk's first human vaccine have spawned international interest in developing a safer AD vaccine and have resulted in a great deal of progress among scientists around the world pursuing this line of research. Animal tests are being used to develop substances that stimulate an immune response without triggering harmful brain inflammation. Investigators are also testing passive immunotherapy strategies, that is, injecting synthetic antibodies against beta-amyloid rather than stimulating the body to produce its own antibodies. Several studies have found that the manufactured beta-amyloid antibodies can remove beta-amyloid plaques and oligomers effectively from the brains of transgenic mice. Studies by a number of groups have shown that antibodies against beta-amyloid can remove beta-amyloid plaques from animals' brains, restore or improve cognition in the animals, and preserve synapses. Other studies have cautioned that tiny blood vessels could be damaged by the method. Scientists are currently working to refine this promising approach.

Dr. Schenk is now involved in human trials of passive immunotherapy with synthetic antibodies genetically engineered to bind specifically to the beta-amyloid peptide; the antibody is called Bapineuzumab and is currently in Phase III of clinical trials. There is also a new, modified version of the vaccine currently in Phase II trials in people with AD. "We give the patients antibodies once every three months, and are assessing whether their thinking improves and whether they can better perform daily functions. We're not finished with the trials yet, but preliminary data from our previous studies are encouraging."

Practical Challenges

Currently, under the FDA guidelines for clinical trials, drugs are tested on people who are already showing symptoms of Alzheimer's disease. Since the desired outcome of any AD drug is improved thinking and memory, researchers measure effectiveness primarily through cognitive testing. However, there is growing apprehension among some scientists regarding whether drugs are being tested on the right population. By the time memory problems emerge, the AD process is well established, so it is possible that a lack of response to a drug may be owing to an advanced disease process rather than an ineffective drug. The memory center of the brain, the hippocampal formation, may be so damaged that it is beyond repair by any drug. Dr. Reisa Sperling conveyed the level of concern many researchers now feel: "The thing that keeps me up at night, the thing that I'm most worried about, is that we're testing these drugs too late in the disease, that once a person already has mild dementia or is at a stage where they've already lost their hippocampal activation, the chances that we can rescue that brain even if we've got a terrific drug and prevent further decline are very small. I think we're going to have a better chance as we move back earlier in the disease to mild cognitive impairment and ultimately perhaps to normal people who have the earliest changes of Alzheimer's disease in their brain. But that's hard."

Dr. John Trojanowski concurred. "The nightmare is that we would eliminate from our arsenal of potential therapeutics drugs that failed in late- or middle-stage Alzheimer's disease—not because they are not potentially disease-modifying or preventative, but because the disease has already wreaked its havoc. It's killed so many cells that there's no therapy that would be efficacious. It would be a terrible loss if those compounds were written off as not being effective because they had shown no efficacy in middle- or late-stage disease. But if used as prevention, they might indeed shut down the disease before it even manifests any symptoms. I don't know the best way to get around that, except to invest more money in research on exactly that question."

Perhaps the most important step needed to expedite the development of preventative drugs is determining a way to accurately and reliably measure the impact of a treatment on the progression of Alzheimer's disease. The only measurements of effectiveness currently recognized by the FDA are clinical and neuropsychological testing, which are subject to great variability since they measure performance that can fluctuate daily. Quantitative measures of biological processes in the body, such as cholesterol levels, are called biomarkers. In the same way that testing a patient's cholesterol can indicate the presence of atherosclerosis or a brain MRI can point to an area where a stroke has occurred, measurements such as beta-amyloid levels in cerebrospinal fluid or PET scans with PiB may be able to identify early pathogenic changes and track the progression of AD. Researchers are at the threshold of determining relationships between biomarkers and AD progression. Once those have been established definitively, scientists will be able to correlate a treatment's effect on a biomarker and its clinical impact on memory or cognitive function as determined by neuropsychological testing. Further research in this area is imperative if any preventative drugs are to be tested on research volunteers determined by these measurements to possess pathology without yet showing symptoms. In order for the FDA to approve the use of any experimental drug in such an ideal test population, investigators will need a way to track the drug's efficacy at preventing the accumulation of pathology or delaying the onset of symptoms.

Dr. Russell Katz, director of the FDA's division of neuropharmacological drug products, described the potential role that biomarkers could play in research on preventative therapies for AD. "There's a lot of interest now in developing treatments for patients who are at risk for the disease but who don't have any symptoms. Everybody's interested in finding a treatment that will prevent the disease or delay the onset of symptoms. That's a very important thing to do. The problem with that approach is that, because the patients don't have symptoms, it's very difficult to know what to measure in order to determine that the drug works. So the question is how you measure the effect of a treatment when you can't measure a patient's symptoms. This is where biomarkers might be useful as indicators that the drug is having an effect on the underlying processes that cause Alzheimer's disease."

Risk and side effects must also be considered. All drugs carry risks of side effects, and some of them can be very serious. As a society we will need to decide what level of risk we are willing to accept to develop aggressive drugs. Speaking for the FDA, Dr. Katz said, "Alzheimer's is a devastating disease. Everybody recognizes that. It's fair to say that as an agency we would be willing to take some risk if we had a drug that really made a profound difference in those patients' lives, or, even better, prevented Alzheimer's disease altogether."

However, these challenges do not dilute the pervasive optimism in the field. As Dr. Sperling told us, "I believe that we've got a cure for Alzheimer's disease in someone's test tube. The question is: how fast can we get that into clinical trials? And do we have the right drugs in clinical trials?" The positive outlook of AD researchers in general, who feel that tremendous progress has been made, was captured by Dr. Aisen: "This is a tremendously exciting time, and we all feel a huge sense of responsibility to work together effectively and get there as fast as we can."

LOOKING FORWARD

Scientists working in the field of Alzheimer's disease research have made incredible strides over the last few decades. A number of the researchers whose work has been featured in this book have described to us the pervasive feeling that now is a time of great promise and momentum in science because of all the knowledge they have accumulated. Tremendous breakthroughs have taken place, and they have traversed an unimaginable distance since Dr. Alois Alzheimer first identified plaques and tangles in 1906.

The incredible talent working on the questions surrounding this complex disease has amassed an impressive number of answers, considering how little was known about AD as recently as the 1980s. Molecular biologists have now identified processes that go awry in the brain to form the hallmark plaques and tangles and interfere with the way brain cells communicate. Geneticists have pinpointed three genes that cause the early-onset form of the disease, as well as the first susceptibility gene that can send people down the path to late-onset AD. Researchers in the field of neuroimaging have progressed from mapping the structure of the brain to measuring brain activity to visualizing the pathology of AD in the living brain through the use of PET scans with PiB compound. Specialists in many of the other conditions that ravage our bodies as we age—from high blood pressure and atherosclerosis to insulin resistance and inflammation—have begun exploring how these problems may act as pathways to AD.

Investigators are applying the knowledge gained through all these different approaches to find drugs that have the potential to postpone or even arrest the development of AD. Researchers may soon understand how the choices we make every day of our lives might alter the blueprints contained in our genes. The field truly is on the threshold not only of understanding this disease, but of understanding how to treat and prevent it.

Until then, however, the research that has already taken place leaves us with a sense of awe—and with an awareness that there are a number of ways we can move forward. Alzheimer's is a horrible disease. There is no diminishing the impact that it has on the individuals who have it and the people who care about and for them. However, those of us who have only lived in fear of it may be able to face it with a new sense of power.

We can take a cue from the front lines of research and work to make our lifestyles as healthy as possible: eating well and exercising regularly; taking steps to prevent high blood pressure, heart disease, and diabetes, or treating those conditions if we already suffer from them; keeping our minds occupied through a lifetime of learning; and staying or becoming engaged in our communities.

We can also take steps to participate in and influence the research that is being carried out today: telling elected representatives that we support funding for this research; giving money ourselves to organizations that sponsor it; volunteering for studies and clinical trials of experimental drugs or lifestyle interventions; or making the ultimate contribution to the field by donating our bodies to science.

The Alzheimer's Project has helped to give us the background, vocabulary, and context to understand the most cutting-edge scientific developments, so that we can keep up with where the field is headed. The more we know about AD, the less there will be to fear.

Still, it's not just people with a relative with AD that are at risk of developing the disease. The most significant risk factor is getting older, and that's certain to happen to all of us, given enough time. Especially as the baby boomers approach retirement age, our entire society is threatened by an explosion of cases of AD. Even if we don't develop the disease ourselves, we are sure to be affected by it as our family and friends age. Until the great minds working to treat or prevent this disease succeed, AD is everyone's problem, which is why we all must become part of the solution.

We asked Dr. Richard Hodes, the director of the National Institute on Aging, why we don't have the answer—today. He assured us: "Science progresses through a succession of discoveries. There's a necessity to have increasing increments of knowledge. This does, unfortunately, limit the speed at which we make progress, and it pains all of us that that's the case. It pains the researchers working in this area, as well as those who see the ravages of the disease. Our commitment, therefore, is to turn from the disappointment we feel at not yet having a cure to a determination to pursue an answer as rapidly as we can, so that we minimize the probability that a few years from now, someone else is going to turn and ask us the very same question: 'Why is it we still don't have the answer?'"

JOHN HOFFMAN AND SUSAN FROEMKE

GLOSSARY

Alzheimer's disease (AD)—a progressive degenerative disease of the brain that causes impairment of memory and other cognitive abilities.

Amnestic—characterized by memory problems; amnestic MCI is a subtype in which memory problems are the most important feature.

Amyloid precursor protein (APP)—the larger protein from which beta-amyloid is formed.

ApoE gene—a gene coding for a protein that carries cholesterol to and within cells; different forms of the ApoE gene are associated with differing risks for late-onset Alzheimer's disease.

Axon—the extension from a neuron that transmits outgoing signals to other neurons.

Beta-amyloid—a part of the amyloid precursor protein found in plaques, the insoluble deposits outside neurons.

Beta-amyloid plaque—a largely insoluble deposit found in the space between nerve cells in the brain. The plaques in Alzheimer's disease are made of beta-amyloid, other molecules, and different kinds of nerve and non-nerve cells.

Blood vessel (capillary)—billions of tiny blood vessels in the brain carry oxygen, glucose (the brain's principal source of energy), nutrients, and hormones like insulin to brain cells so they can do their work, and remove carbon dioxide and cell waste products.

Blood-brain barrier—a barrier that prevents most large molecules, red and white blood cells, and disease-causing organisms (such as bacteria) in the bloodstream from moving into the brain. The barrier is formed by a type of glial cell aided by tight junctions that act like little "spot welds" between adjacent endothelial cells that constitute the lining of brain blood vessels.

Brain-derived neurotrophic factor (BDNF)—a growth factor that stimulates survival, growth, and adaptability of some neurons.

Cerebral cortex—the outermost layer of the cerebral hemispheres sometimes referred to as the gray matter. It is composed of neurons and nerve fibers and associated support cells called glia.

Cerebrospinal fluid—the fluid found in and around the brain and spinal cord. One of its functions is to cushion the brain hydraulically.

Chromosome—this thread-like structure in the nucleus of a cell contains DNA. DNA sequences make up genes. Most human cells have twenty-three pairs of chromosomes containing approximately thirty thousand genes.

Clinical trial—a research study involving humans; rigorously tests safety, side effects, and the effectiveness of a medication or behavioral treatment.

Cognition—conscious thought and mental activity, including learning, perceiving, making decisions, and remembering.

Dementia—a broad term referring to a decline in cognitive function that interferes with daily life and activities.

Dendrite—a branch-like extension of a neuron that receives messages from other neurons.

Diabetes—chronic metabolic disorder in which the body doesn't produce or properly use insulin, a hormone that is made in the pancreas and is essential for the healthy functioning of all cells in the body.

DNA (deoxyribonucleic acid)—DNA forms two long, intertwined, thread-like strands called chromosomes. Each cell has 46 chromosomes in 23 pairs, which are found in the nucleus. The DNA in chromosomes is made up of four chemicals, or bases, strung together in various sequence patterns. The DNA in nearly all cells of an individual is identical. Each chromosome contains many thousands of segments, called genes.

Early-onset Alzheimer's disease—a rare form of AD that usually affects people between ages thirty and sixty. It is called familial AD (FAD) if it runs in the family.

Entorhinal cortex—an area within the brain where damage from AD often begins.

Epidemiological study—a study of the causes, distribution, and control of disease in populations, with emphasis on investigating relationships between personal characteristics (demographic, socioeconomic, lifestyle, biological, and genetic) and occurrence of disease.

Enzyme—a protein that causes or speeds up a biochemical reaction.

Free radical—a highly reactive molecule (typically oxygen or nitrogen) that combines easily with other molecules because it contains an unpaired electron. The combination with other molecules sometimes damages cells.

Functional MRI (fMRI)—an adaptation of an MRI imaging technique that measures brain activity during a mental task, such as one involving memory, language, or attention.

Gene—the biologic unit of heredity passed from parent to child. Genes are segments of DNA and contain instructions that tell a cell how to make specific proteins.

Genetic risk factor—a variant in a cell's DNA that does not cause a disease by itself but may increase the chance that a person will develop a disease.

Glial cell—a type of brain cell that supports, protects, or nourishes neurons.

Hippocampal formation—a structure in the brain that plays a major role in learning and memory and is involved in converting short-term to long-term memory.

Inflammation—the process by which the body responds to cellular injury by attempting to eliminate foreign matter and damaged tissue.

Insulin resistance—a condition in which the pancreas makes enough insulin, but the cells do not respond properly to it; characterizes and precedes type 2 diabetes.

Late-onset Alzheimer's disease—the most common form of AD. It occurs in people aged sixty and older.

Magnetic resonance imaging (MRI)—a diagnostic and research technique that uses magnetic fields to generate a computer image of internal structures in the body.

Metabolism—all the chemical processes that take place inside the body. In some metabolic reactions, complex molecules are broken down to release energy. In others, the cells use energy to make complex compounds out of simpler ones (like making proteins from amino acids).

Microtubule—an internal support structure for a neuron that guides organelles and molecules from the body of the cell to the end of the axon.

Mild cognitive impairment (MCI)—a condition in which a person has memory problems greater than those expected for his or her age, but not the personality or other cognitive problems that characterize AD.

Mutation—a permanent change in the DNA of a cell that can affect the structure of a protein to such an extent that it causes a disease.

Myelin—Whitish layers of compacted glial cell membranes that surround and insulate an axon, allowing the axon to transmit electrical messages more rapidly from the cell body to the synapse.

Neurodegenerative disease—a disease characterized by a progressive decline in the structure, activity, and function of brain tissue. These diseases include AD, Parkinson's disease, frontotemporal lobar degeneration, and dementia with Lewy bodies. They are usually more common in older people.

Neurofibrillary tangle—a collection of twisted and hyperphosphorylated tau found in the cell body, axons, and dendrites of a neuron in AD.

Neuron—a nerve cell.

Neurotransmitter—a chemical messenger between neurons. These substances are released by the axon on one neuron and excite or inhibit activity in a neighboring neuron.

Nonamnestic—not characterized by memory problems; nonamnestic MCI is characterized by a decline in other cognitive skills, and is not thought to be an early stage of Alzheimer's disease.

Nucleus—the structure within a cell that contains the chromosomes and controls many of its activities.

Oligomers—clusters of a small number of beta-amyloid peptides.

Oxidative damage—damage that can occur to cells when they are exposed to too many free radicals.

Pathology—structural and functional changes that result from a disease process.

Pittsburgh Compound B (PiB)—the radioactive tracer compound used during a PET scan of the brain to show beta-amyloid deposits.

Positron emission tomography (PET)—an imaging technique using radioisotopes that allows researchers to observe and measure activity in different parts of the brain by monitoring blood flow and concentrations of substances such as oxygen and glucose, as well as other specific constituents of brain tissues.

Susceptibility gene—see genetic risk factor.

Synapse—the tiny gap between nerve cells across which neurotransmitters pass.

Tau—a protein that helps to maintain the structure of microtubules in normal nerve cells. Abnormal tau is a principal component of the paired helical filaments in neurofibrillary tangles.

Transgenic—an animal that has had a gene (like human APP) inserted into its chromosomes. Mice carrying a mutated human APP gene often develop plaques in their brains as they age.

TO LEARN MORE

The Alzheimer's Project

This book is part of The Alzheimer's Project, a multi-platform public health initiative. The project's four documentary films premiered on HBO from May 10–12, 2009. Those films, along with twelve supplemental films, are available for purchase on DVD, in addition to being available free of charge on HBO.com, YouTube, and iTunes.

Alzheimer's Disease Education and Referral (ADEAR) Center
National Institute on Aging
National Institutes of Health
U.S. Department of Health and Human Services
P.O. Box 8250
Silver Spring, MD 20907-8250
800-438-4380 (toll-free)
www.nia.nih.gov/Alzheimers

This service of the federal government's National Institute on Aging (NIA) offers information and publications on diagnosis, treatment, patient care, caregiver needs, long-term care, education and training, and research related to Alzheimer's disease. Staff members answer telephone, e-mail, and written requests, and make referrals to local and national resources. The ADEAR Web site offers free online publications in English and Spanish; e-mail alerts and online Connections newsletter registration; an AD clinical trials database; the AD Library data-base; and a listing of the NIA's Alzheimer's disease research centers around the United States, and more.

Alzheimer's Association
225 North Michigan Avenue
Suite 1700
Chicago, IL 60601-7633
800-272-3900 (toll-free)
www.alz.org

The Alzheimer's Association is the leading voluntary health organization in Alzheimer care, support, and research. The Alzheimer's Association delivers education, support, and services for people diagnosed with Alzheimer's disease, their families, caregivers, healthcare professionals, and the general public. Programs delivered at the nationwide level include a twenty-four-hour helpline for information and referrals, online education, and assistance at www.alz.org, housing- and care-finder services, an identification program designed to address wandering and to return people home safely, and nationwide campaigns about the warning signs of Alzheimer's disease, risk reduction, and the effects of the disease on the brain. A network of local chapters sponsors support groups and educational programs, and offers referrals to local resources and services. A wide variety of online and print publications and videos are also available. The association is the leading nonprofit funder of Alzheimer's disease research.

Additional Resources

Alzheimer's Disease Cooperative Study
858-622-5880
http://adcs.ucsd.edu

The Alzheimer's Disease Cooperative Study (ADCS) is a cooperative agreement between the National Institute on Aging and the University of California San Diego to advance research in the development of drugs to treat AD. The ADCS is a consortium of medical research centers and clinics working to develop clinical trials of medicines to treat behavioral symptoms, improve cognition, slow the rate of decline, delay the onset, or prevent Alzheimer's disease altogether. The ADCS also develops new and more reliable ways to evaluate patients enrolled in clinical trials.

Alzheimer's Drug Discovery Foundation (ADDF)
www.alzdiscovery.org

The ADDF is an affiliated public charity of the Institute for the Study of Aging funding drug discovery research for Alzheimer's disease, related dementias, and cognitive aging.

Alzheimer's Foundation of America
866-232-8484 (toll-free)
www.alzfdn.org

The Alzheimer's Foundation of America provides care and services to individuals confronting dementia and to their caregivers and families, through member organizations dedicated to improving quality of life. Services include a toll-free hotline, consumer publications and other educational materials, and conferences and workshops.

Alzheimer Research Forum
www.alzforum.org

The Alzheimer Research Forum, an online community and resource center, offers professionals and the general public access to an annotated index of scientific papers, research news, moderated discussions on scientific topics, libraries of animal models and antibodies, and directories of clinical trials, conferences, jobs, and research-funding sources.

American Academy of Neurology
800-879-1960 (toll-free) or 651-695-2717
www.aan.com
www.thebrainmatters.org

The American Academy of Neurology (AAN) is an international professional association of neurologists and neuroscience professionals dedicated to providing the best possible care for patients with neurological disorders. In addition to providing services for its members, AAN provides referrals to neurologists who are members. The AAN Foundation also produces educational materials for the public, including the Web site "The Brain Matters," which seeks to explain common disorders of the brain including AD. Publications for the public include a free patient magazine, updates from *Neurology*, and guidelines that summarize research on recognizing, diagnosing, and providing treatment options for people with AD and their families.

American Health Assistance Foundation
1-800-437-AHAF
www.ahaf.org

The American Health Assistance Foundation (AHAF) is a nonprofit organization that funds research seeking cures for Alzheimer's disease and age-related macular degeneration and glaucoma, and provides the public with information about risk factors, the latest research, treatments, risk reduction through healthy lifestyles, and ways to cope with the effects of these diseases.

Children of Aging Parents
800-227-7294 (toll-free)
www.caps4caregivers.org

This nonprofit organization provides information and referrals for nursing homes, retirement communities, elder law attorneys, adult day care centers, insurance providers, respite care, assisted living centers, support groups, and state and county agencies. It also offers fact sheets, a newsletter, and conferences and workshops.

ClinicalTrials.gov
www.ClinicalTrials.gov

ClinicalTrials.gov is an online registry of federally and privately supported clinical trials conducted in the United States and around the world. Users can search for clinical trials and find information about each trial's purpose, who may participate, locations, and phone numbers for more details.

Dana Alliance for Brain Initiatives
212-223-4040
www.dana.org/danaalliances

The Dana Alliance for Brain Initiatives, a nonprofit organization of more than 265 leading neuroscientists, helps advance public awareness about the progress and promise of brain research and disseminates information about the brain. The Dana Alliance sponsors "Brain Awareness Week" each year, and provides teaching resources and other materials for the public.

Eldercare Locator
800-677-1116 (toll-free)
www.eldercare.gov

Eldercare Locator is a nationwide, directory assistance service helping older people and their caregivers locate local support and resources. It is sponsored by the U.S. Administration on Aging at the Department of Health and Human Services, whose Web site at www.aoa.gov also features Alzheimer's disease information for families, caregivers, and health professionals.

Family Caregiver Alliance
800-445-8106 (toll-free)
www.caregiver.org

The Family Caregiver Alliance is a nonprofit organization that offers support services and information for people caring for adults with Alzheimer's disease, stroke, traumatic brain injuries, and other cognitive disorders.

MedlinePlus
National Library of Medicine
National Institutes of Health
U.S. Department of Health and Human Services
www.nlm.nih.gov/medlineplus

MedlinePlus brings together the resources of the world's largest medical library, The National Library of Medicine, in a format designed for the general public. There are directories; a medical encyclopedia and a medical dictionary; easy-to-understand tutorials on common conditions, tests, and treatments; health information in Spanish; extensive information on prescription and nonprescription drugs; health information from the media; and links to clinical trials.

National Academy of Elder Law Attorneys (NAELA)
703-942-5711
www.naela.org

The National Academy of Elder Law Attorneys is a nonprofit association that assists lawyers, bar organizations, and others who work with older clients and their families. The academy provides a resource of information, education, networking, and assistance to those who deal with the many specialized issues involved with legal services to seniors and people with special needs.

National Cell Repository for Alzheimer's Disease (NCRAD)
800-526-2839
www.ncrad.org

NCRAD is a National Institute on Aging–funded national resource where clinical information and genetic material (DNA) from individuals with Alzheimer's disease, as well as from individuals without any symptoms of memory loss or dementia, can be stored. NCRAD is part of a new effort to help researchers identify the genes that play a role in the development of Alzheimer's disease. Contact NCRAD for information about ongoing AD genetics studies.

National Family Caregivers Association

800-896-3650 (toll-free)
301-942-6430
www.thefamilycaregiver.org

The National Family Caregivers Association helps educate and support people who care for loved ones with chronic illness, disability, or the frailties of old age. The association offers an online library of information and educational materials, workshops, and other resources.

National Hospice and Palliative Care Organization

800-658-8898 (toll-free)
www.nhpco.org

This nonprofit organization works to enhance the quality of life for people who are terminally ill. It provides information, resources, and referrals to local hospice services, and offers publications and online resources.

National Long Term Care Ombudsman Resource Center

http://www.ltcombudsman.org

The center, supported by a grant from the Administration on Aging, seeks to enhance the lives of long-term care residents by supporting the work of state ombudsmen (citizen representatives). They advocate for residents' rights and quality care, educate consumers and providers, work to resolve residents' complaints, and provide information to the public. You can search a map of the United States on their Web site to find ombudsmen in your state.

Society for Neuroscience

202-962-4000
www.sfn.org

The Society for Neuroscience (SfN) is a nonprofit membership organization of scientists and physicians who study the brain and nervous system. The society also promotes public information and general education about the nature of scientific discovery and the results and implications of the latest neuroscience research, and produces a variety of publications, including a monthly newsletter and a primer on the brain and nervous system.

Well Spouse Association

800-838-0879 (toll-free)
www.wellspouse.org

The nonprofit Well Spouse Association gives support to spouses and partners of people who are chronically ill and/or disabled. It offers support groups and a newsletter.

INDEX

The index for this book is available online at www.publicaffairsbooks.com/HBO.pdf

PUBLICAFFAIRS is a publishing house founded in 1997. It is a tribute to the standards, values, and flair of three persons who have served as mentors to countless reporters, writers, editors, and book people of all kinds, including me.

I. F. STONE, proprietor of *I. F. Stone's Weekly,* combined a commitment to the First Amendment with entrepreneurial zeal and reporting skill and became one of the great independent journalists in American history. At the age of eighty, Izzy published *The Trial of Socrates,* which was a national bestseller. He wrote the book after he taught himself ancient Greek.

BENJAMIN C. BRADLEE was for nearly thirty years the charismatic editorial leader of *The Washington Post.* It was Ben who gave the *Post* the range and courage to pursue such historic issues as Watergate. He supported his reporters with a tenacity that made them fearless, and it is no accident that so many became authors of influential, best-selling books.

ROBERT L. BERNSTEIN, the chief executive of Random House for more than a quarter century, guided one of the nation's premier publishing houses. Bob was personally responsible for many books of political dissent and argument that challenged tyranny around the globe. He is also the founder and was the longtime chair of Human Rights Watch, one of the most respected human rights organizations in the world.

· · ·

For fifty years, the banner of Public Affairs Press was carried by its owner Morris B. Schnapper, who published Gandhi, Nasser, Toynbee, Truman, and about 1,500 other authors. In 1983 Schnapper was described by *The Washington Post* as "a redoubtable gadfly." His legacy will endure in the books to come.

Peter Osnos, *Founder and Editor-at-Large*